Published by
Nature Photobook Publishing

The following 40 photographs have been specially selected to promote relaxation.

Enjoy beautiful island photographs taken in Barbados:

- Beaches
- Colorful tropical flowers
- Birds and animals

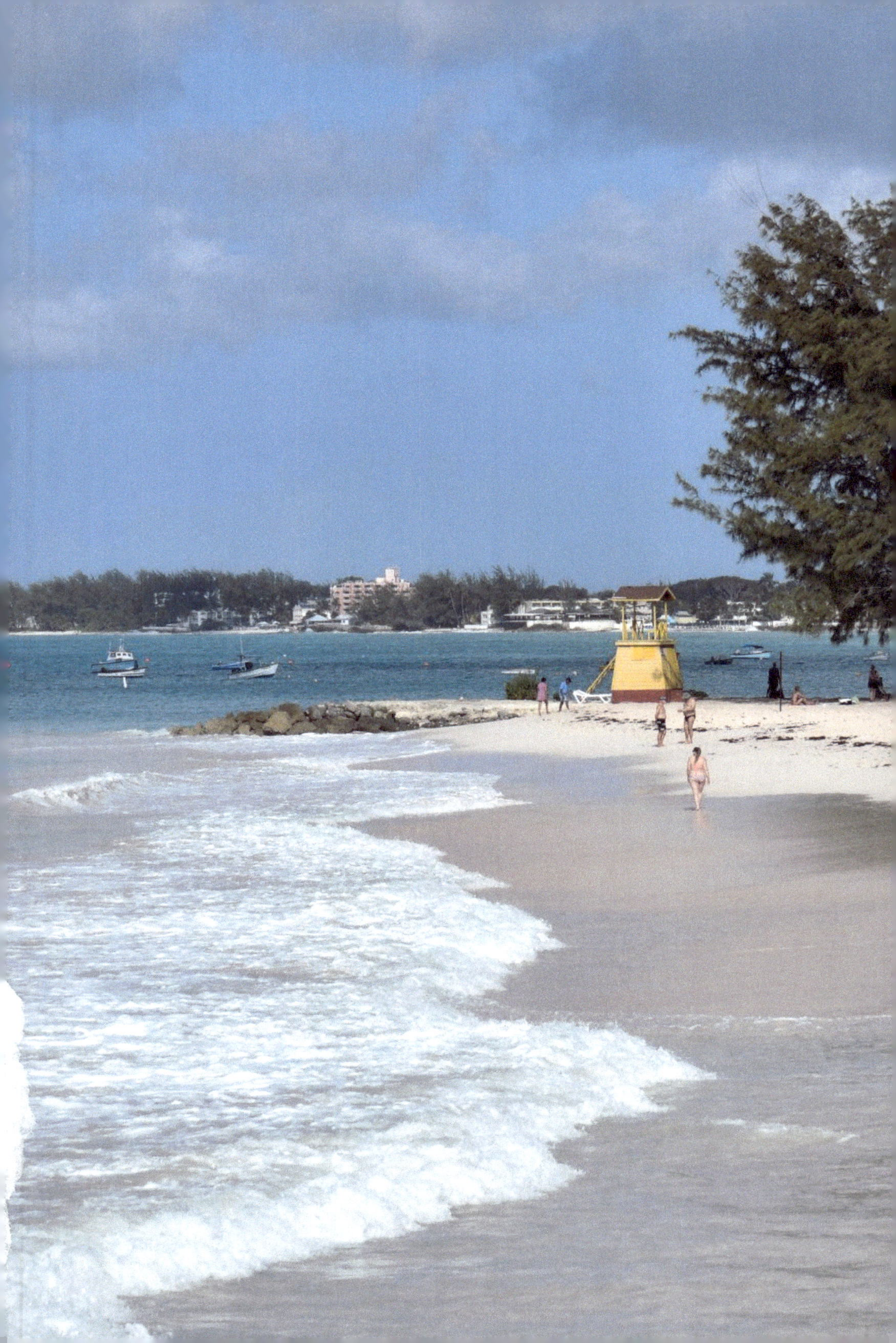

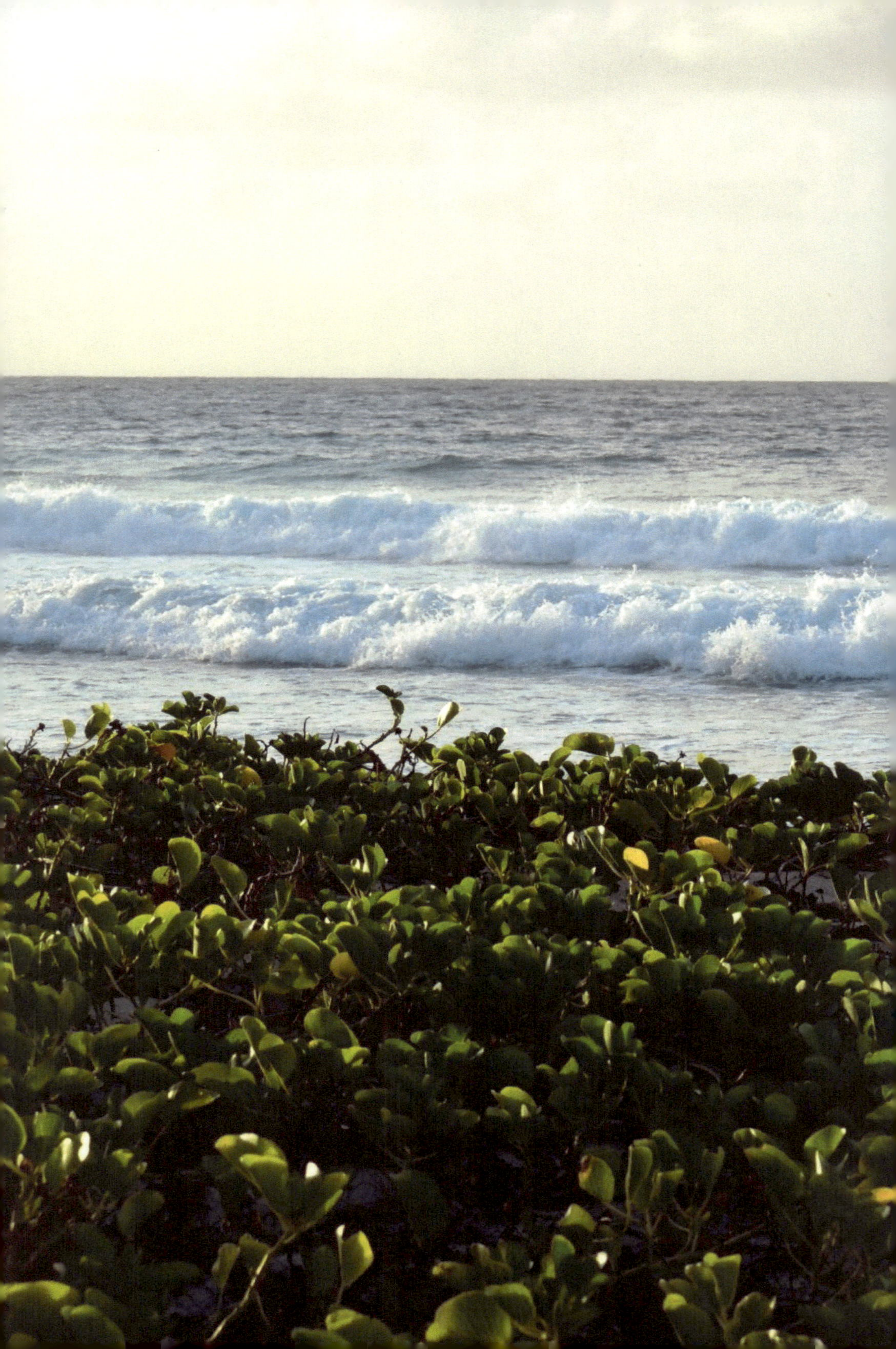

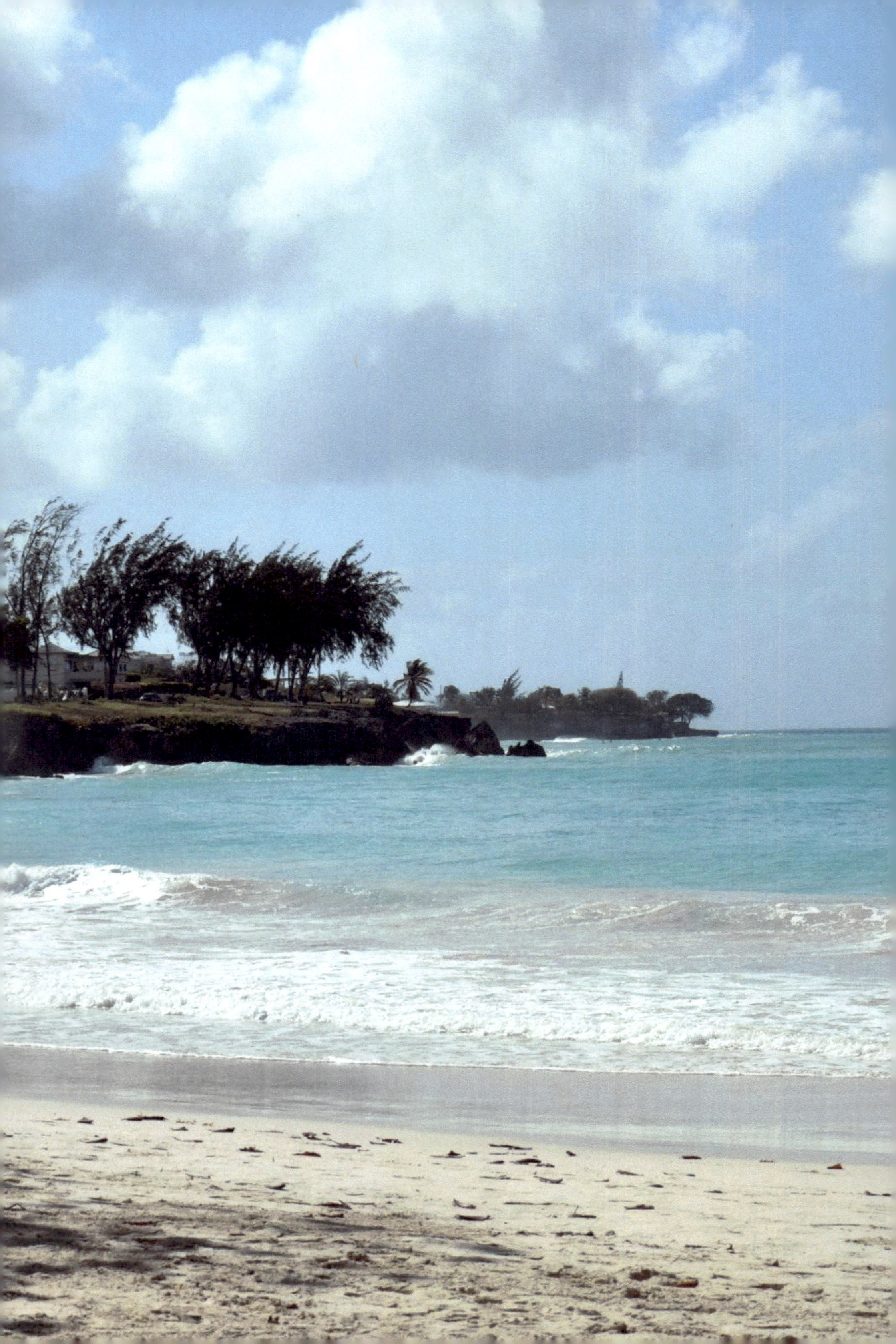

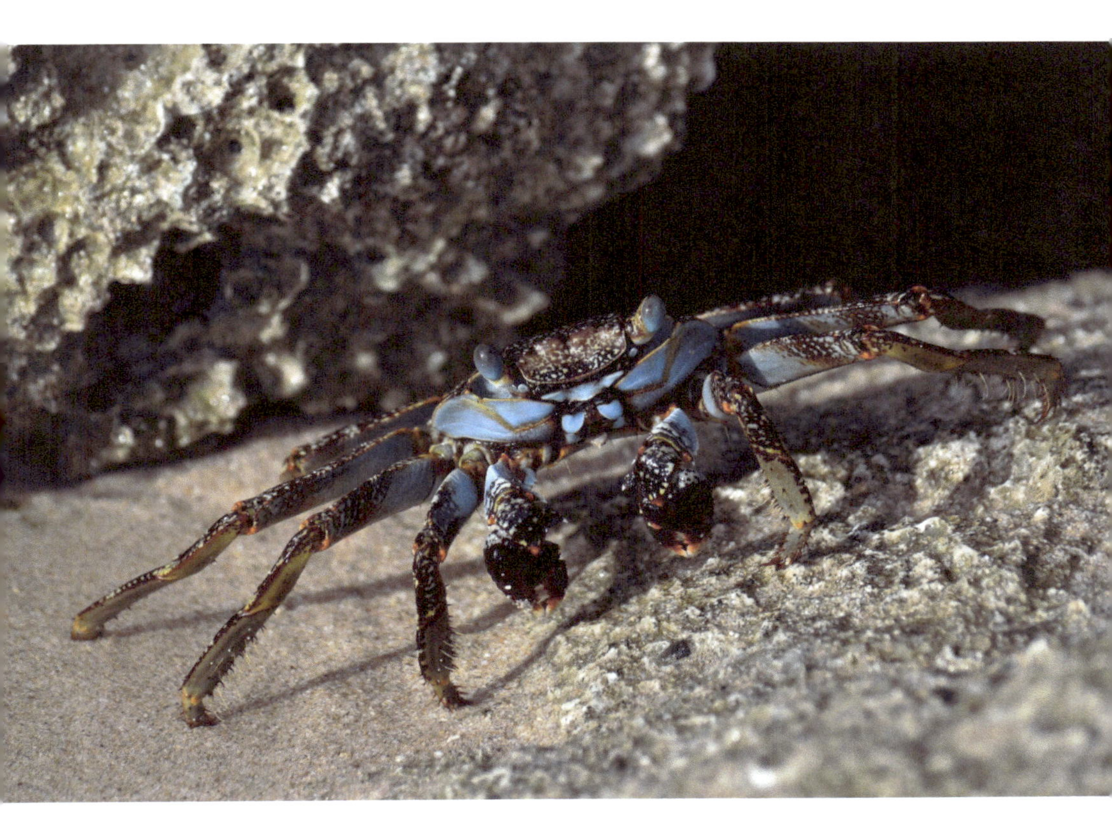

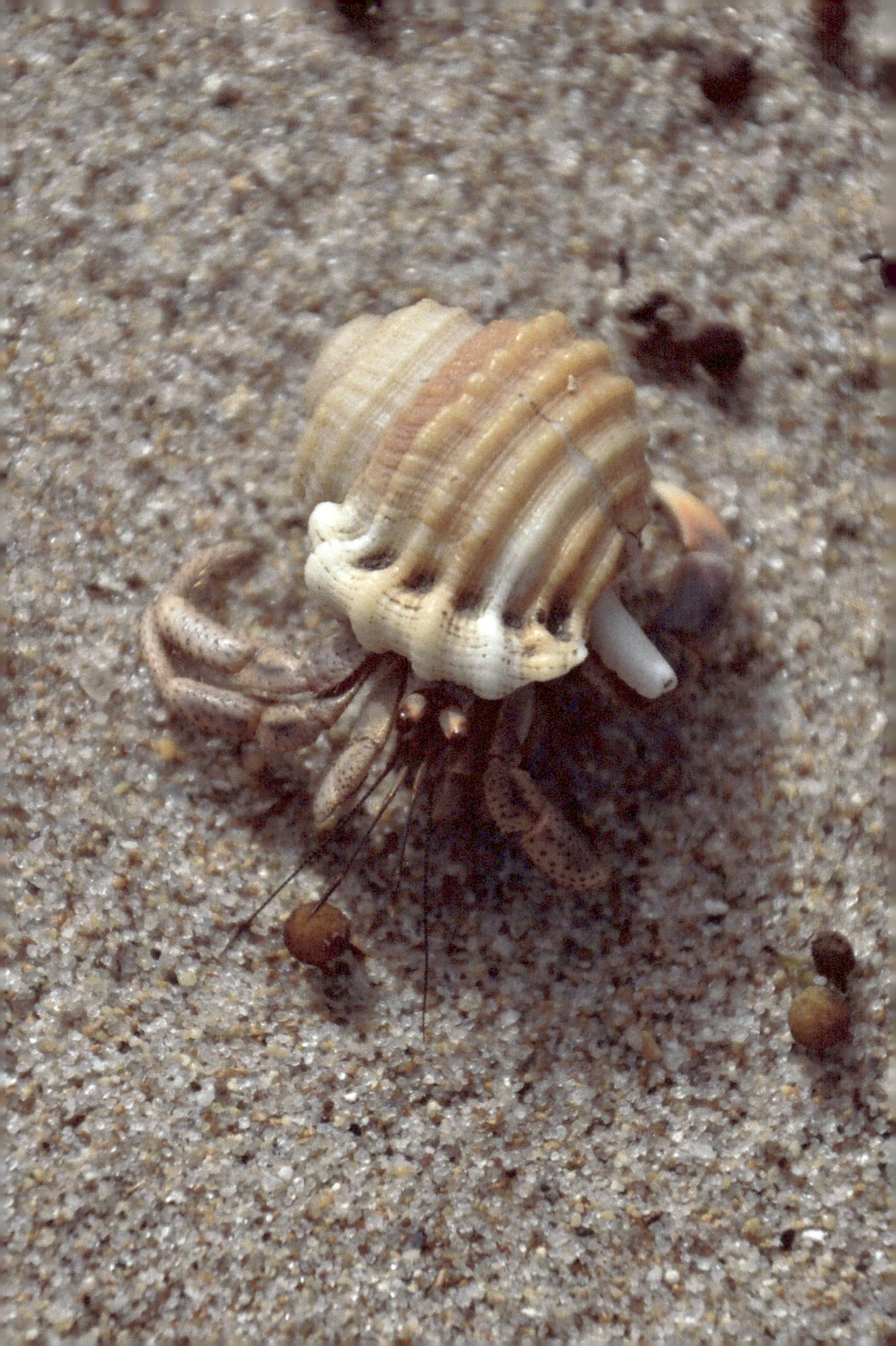

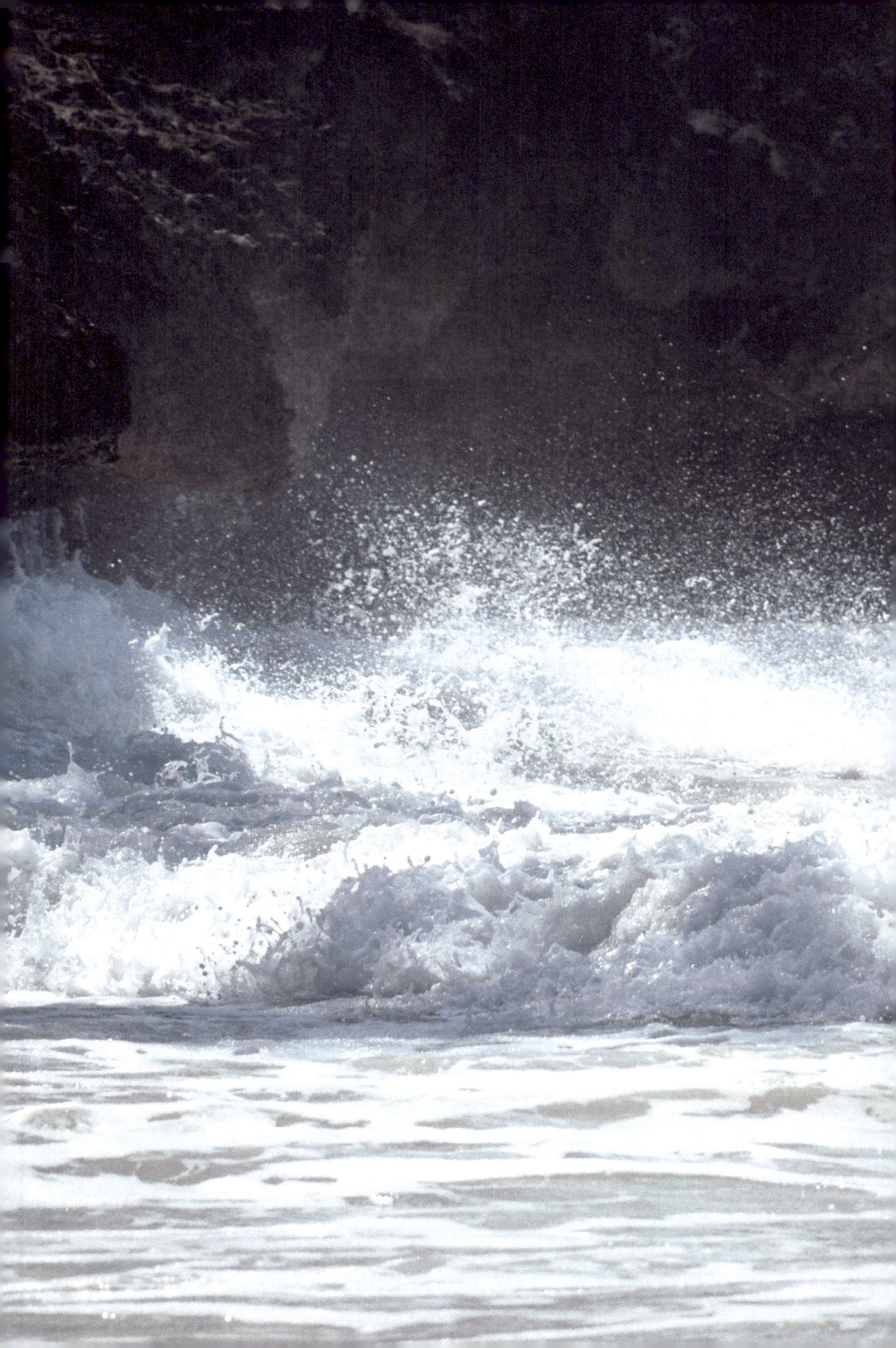

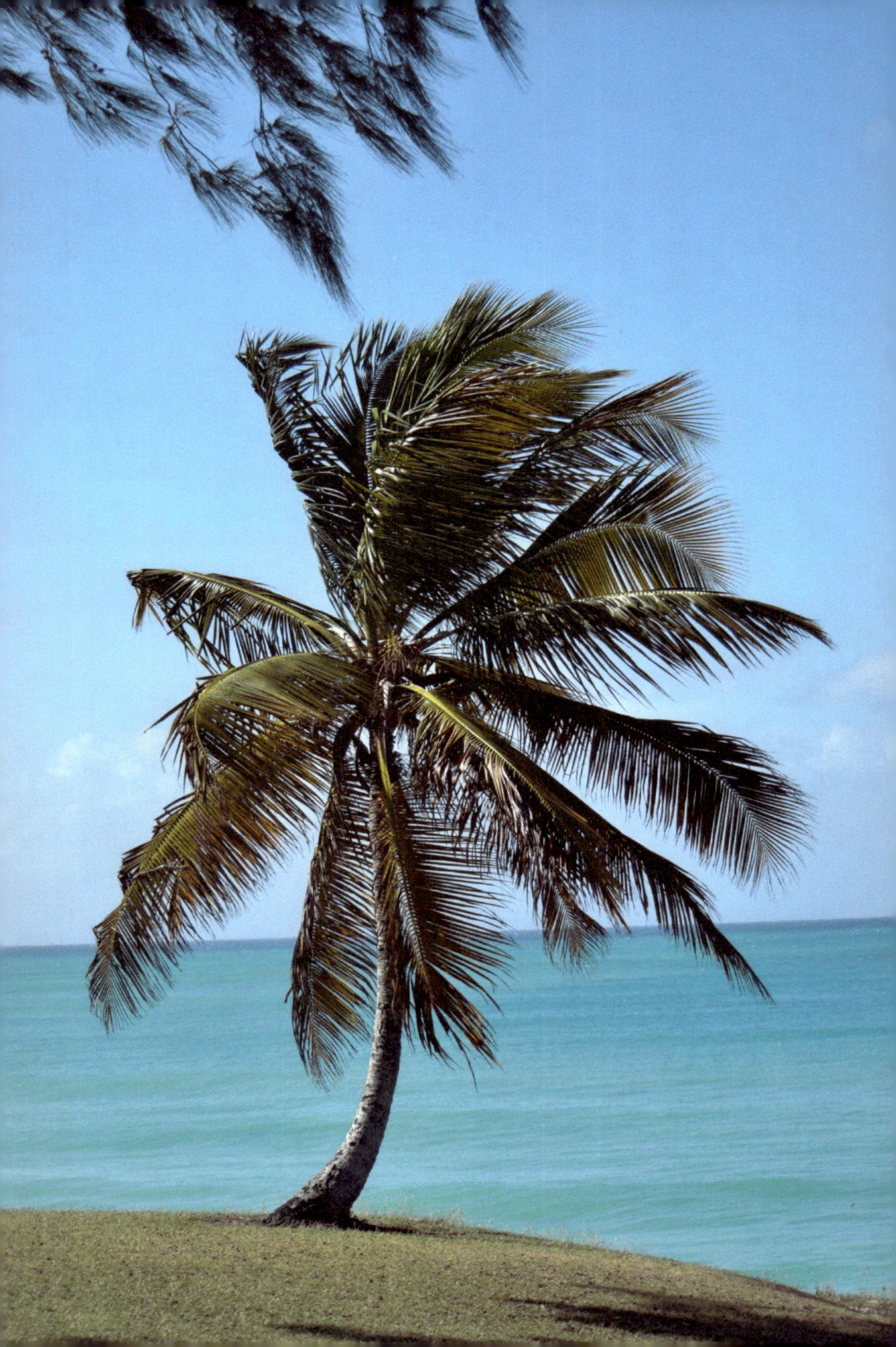

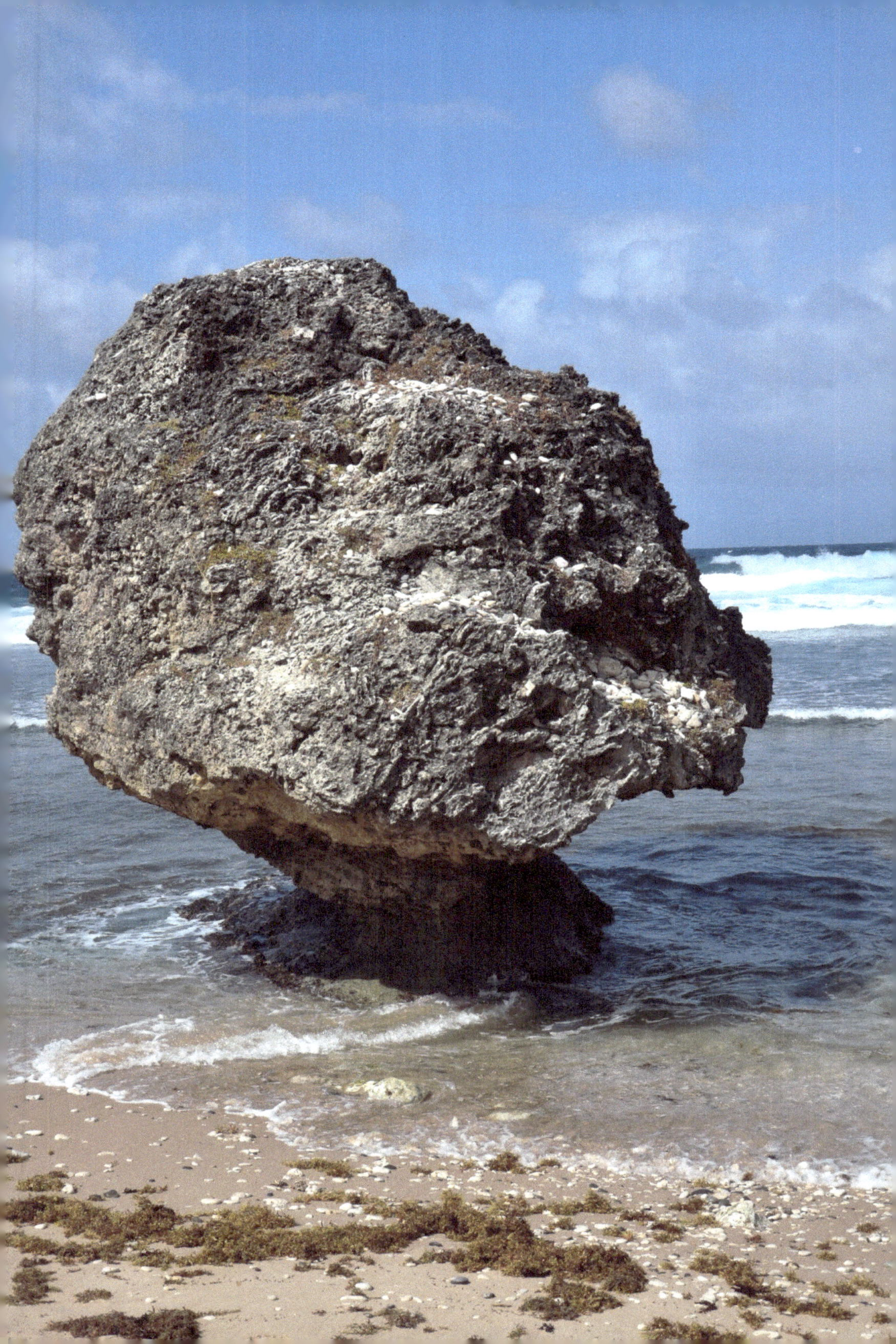

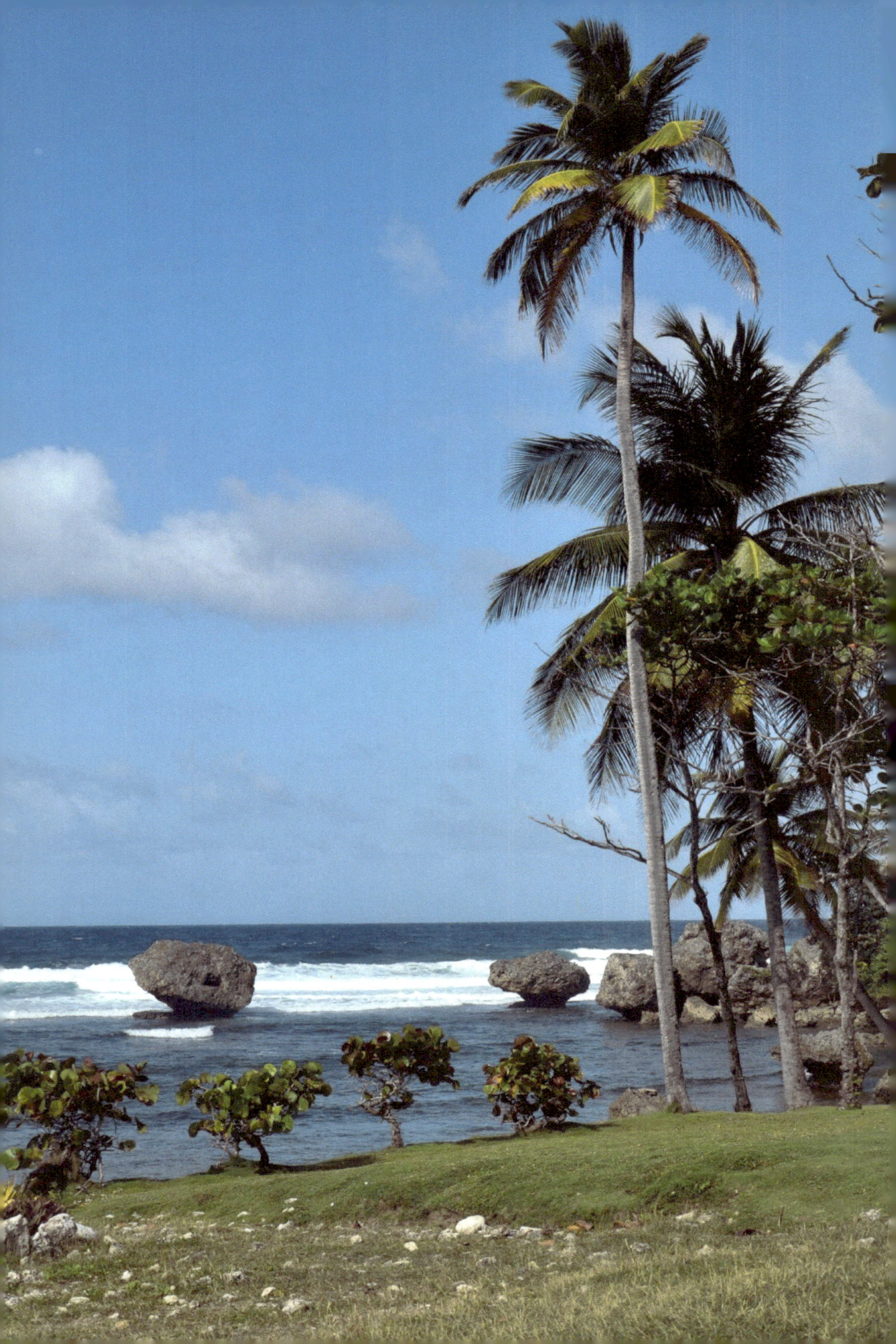

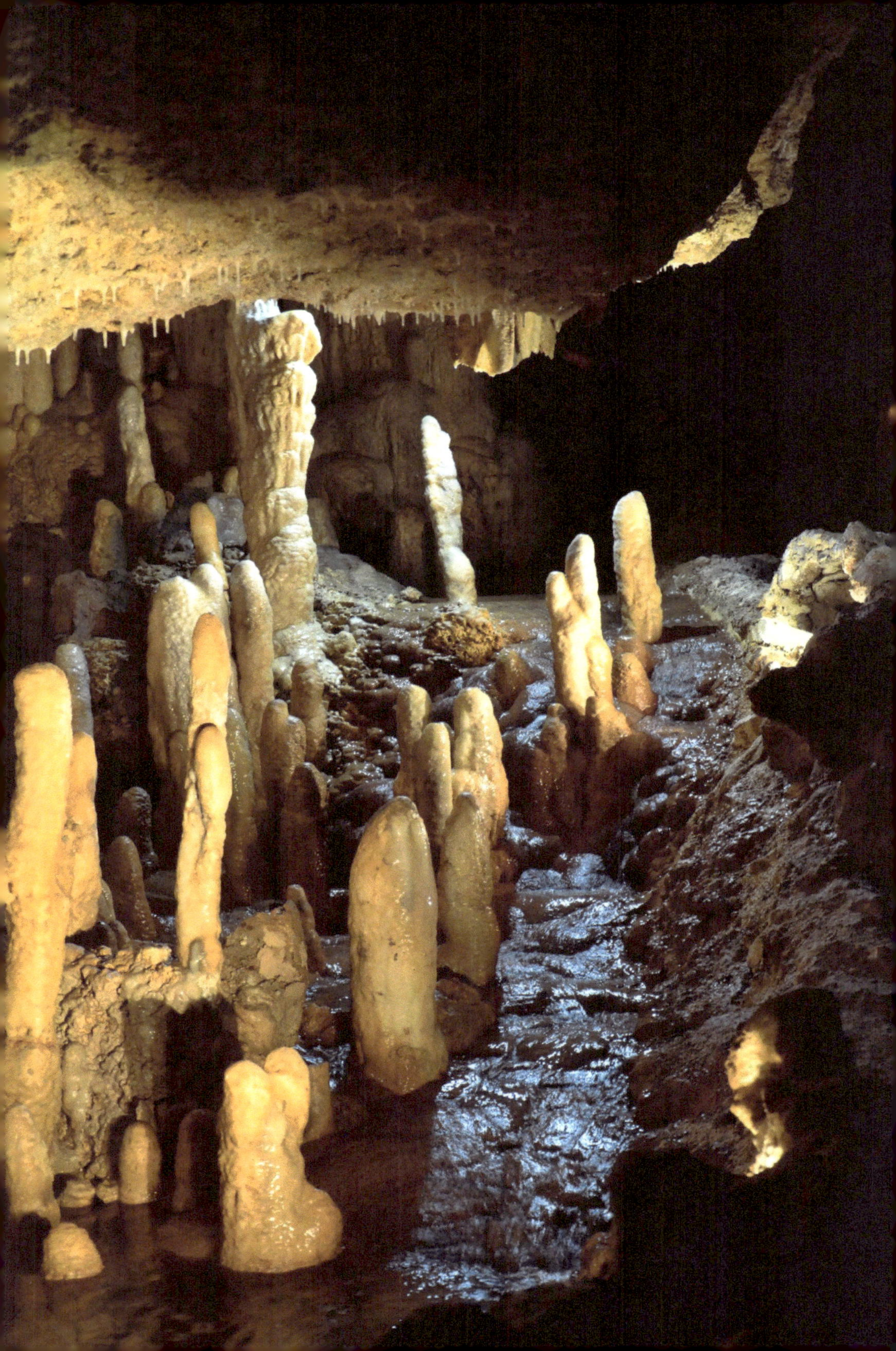

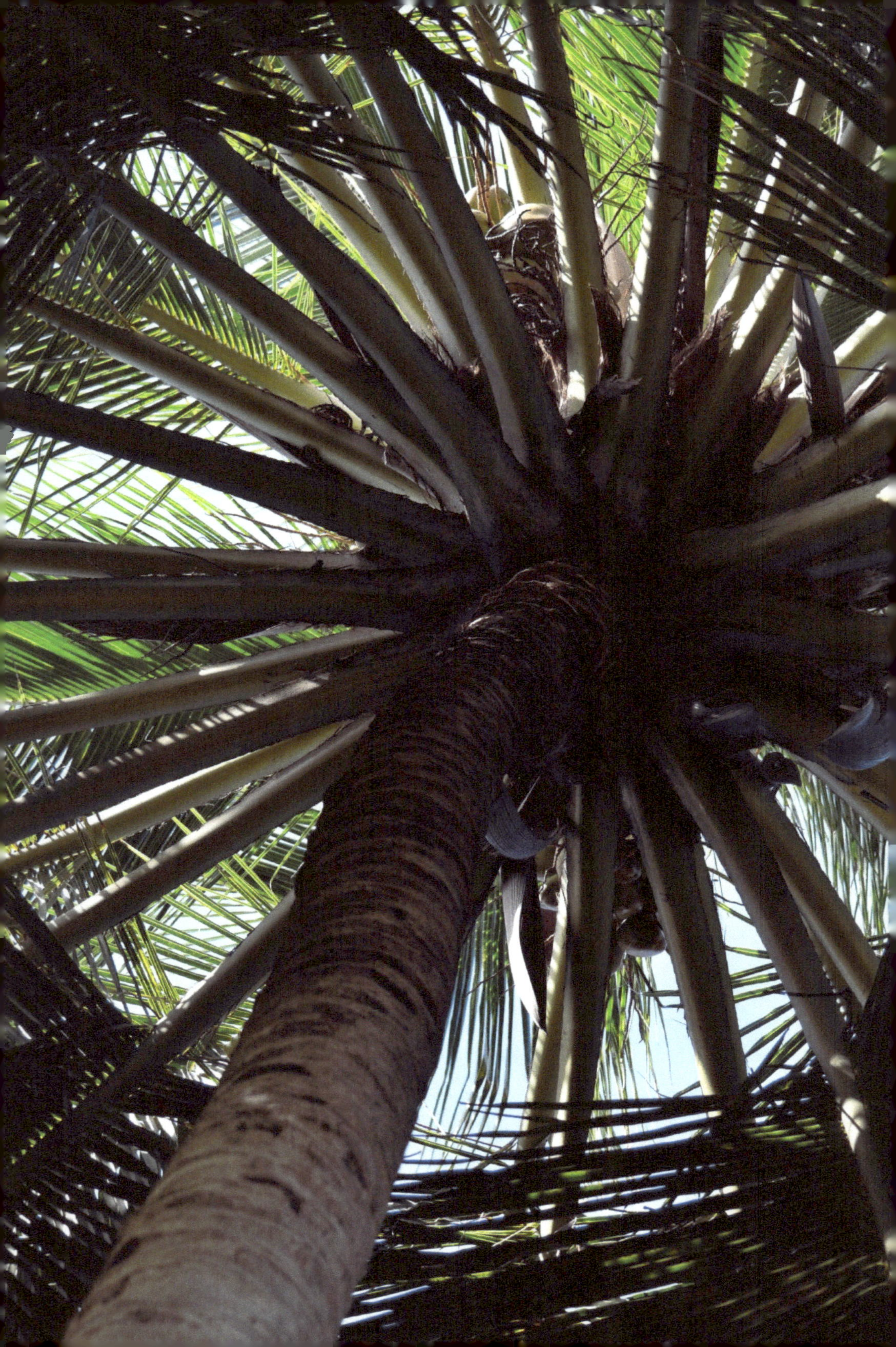

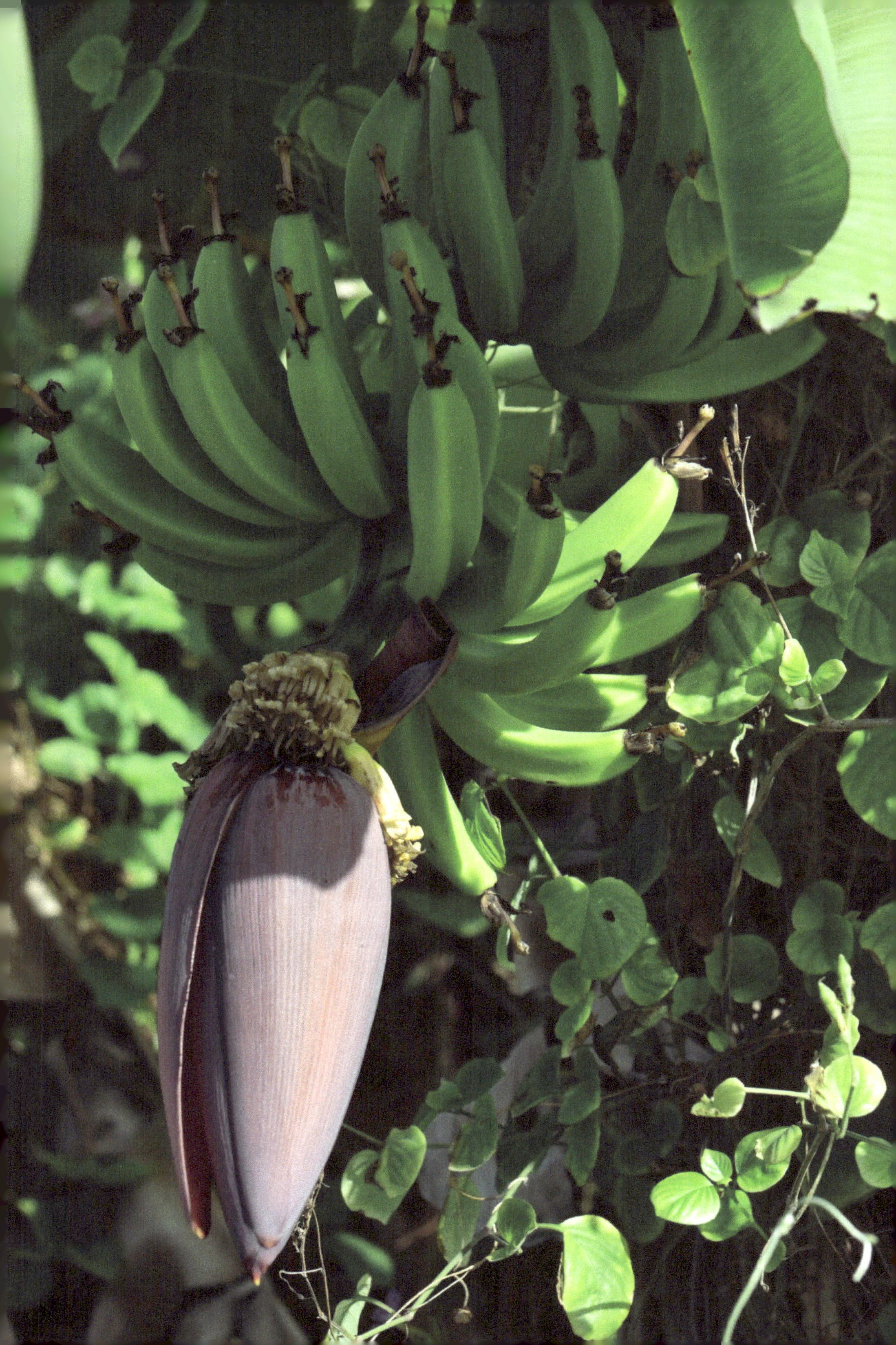

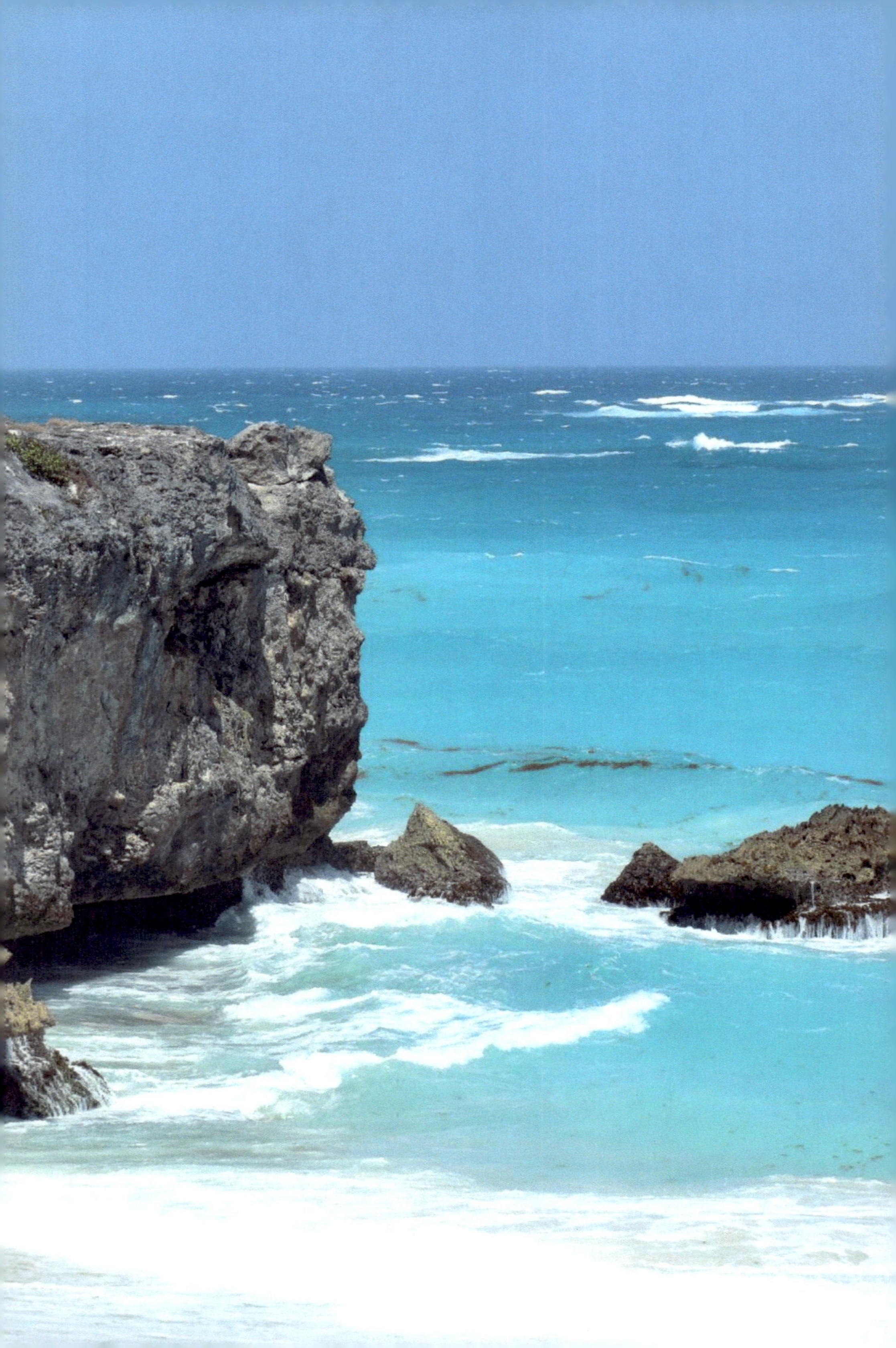

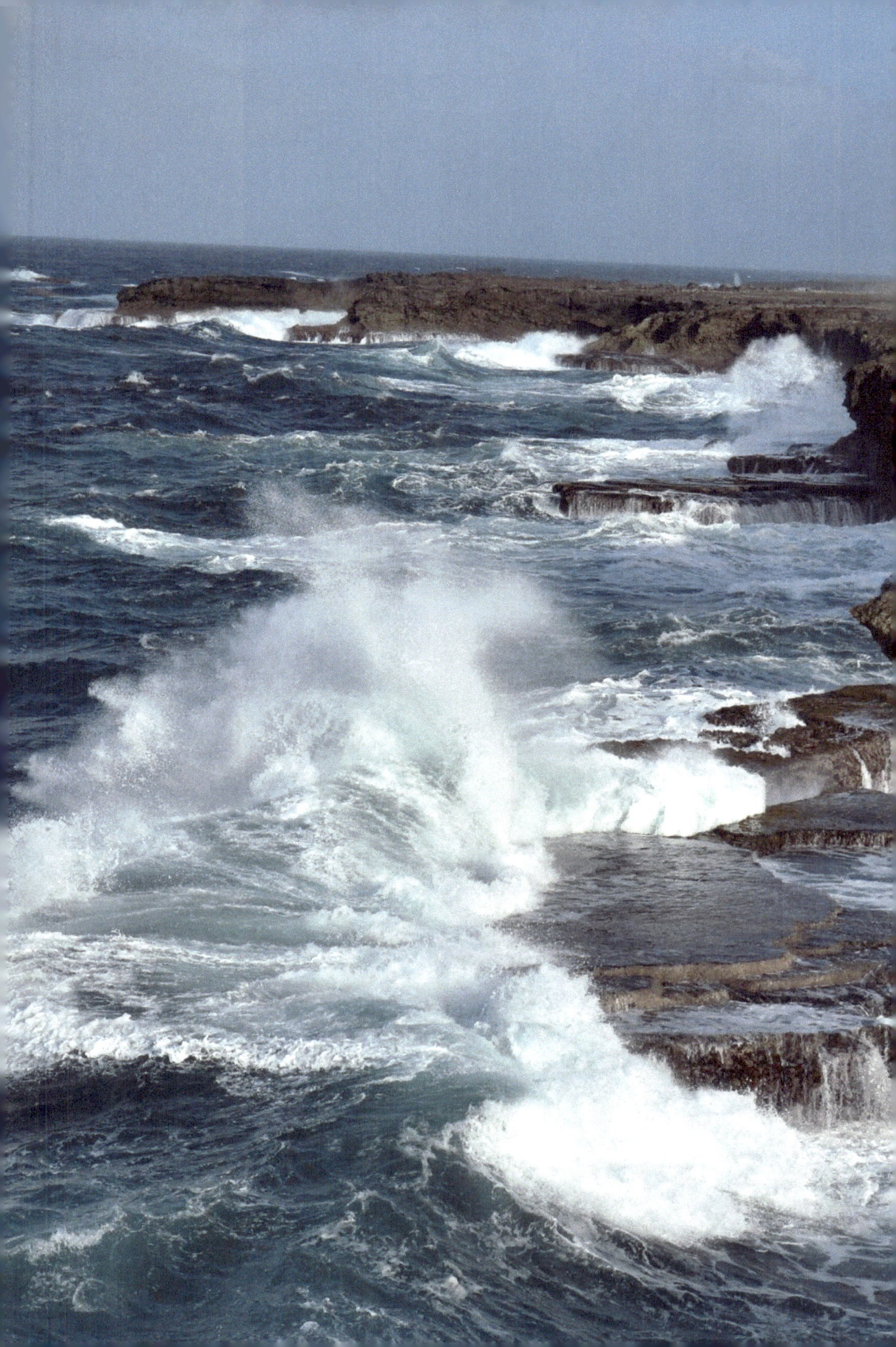

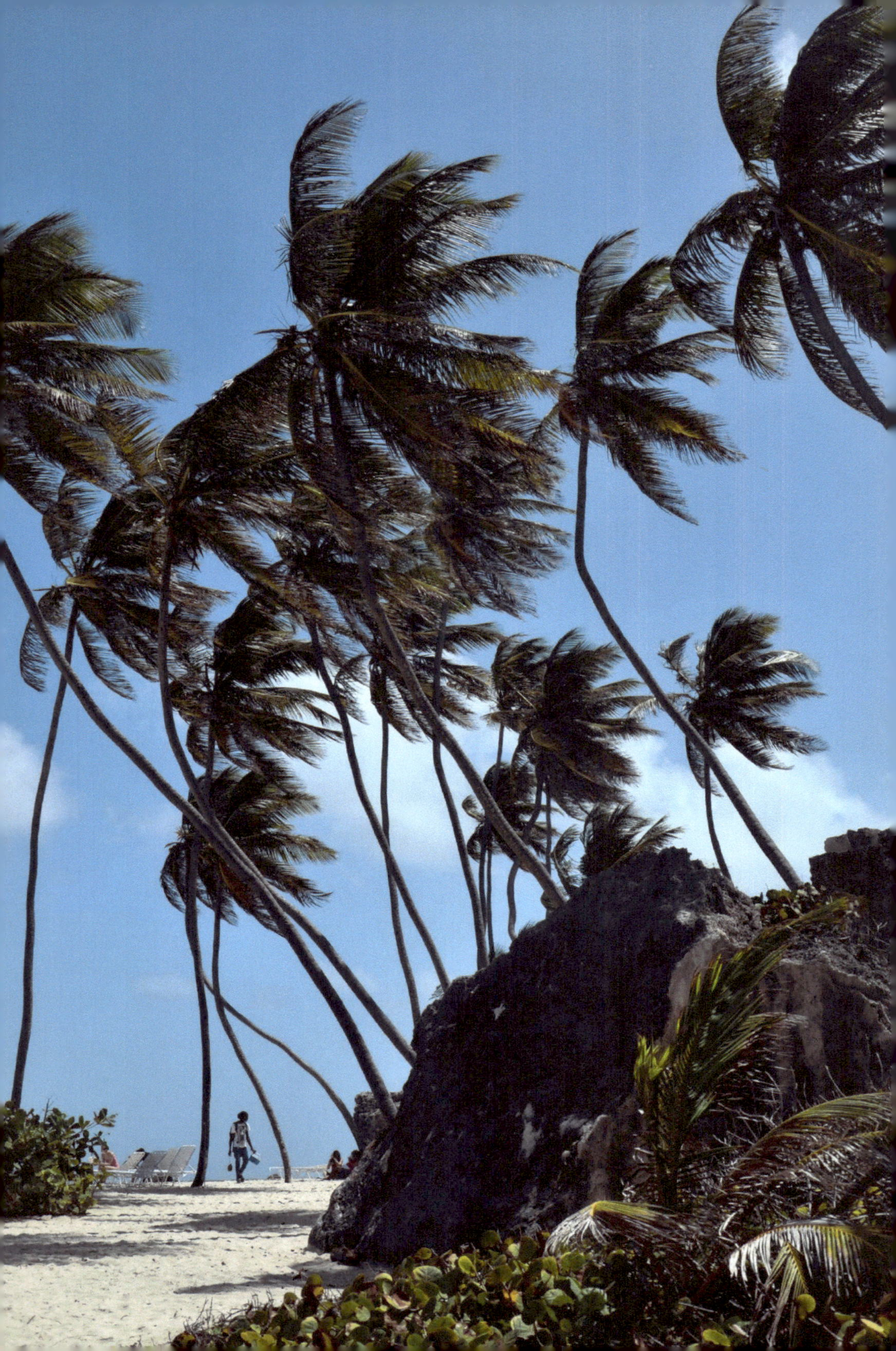

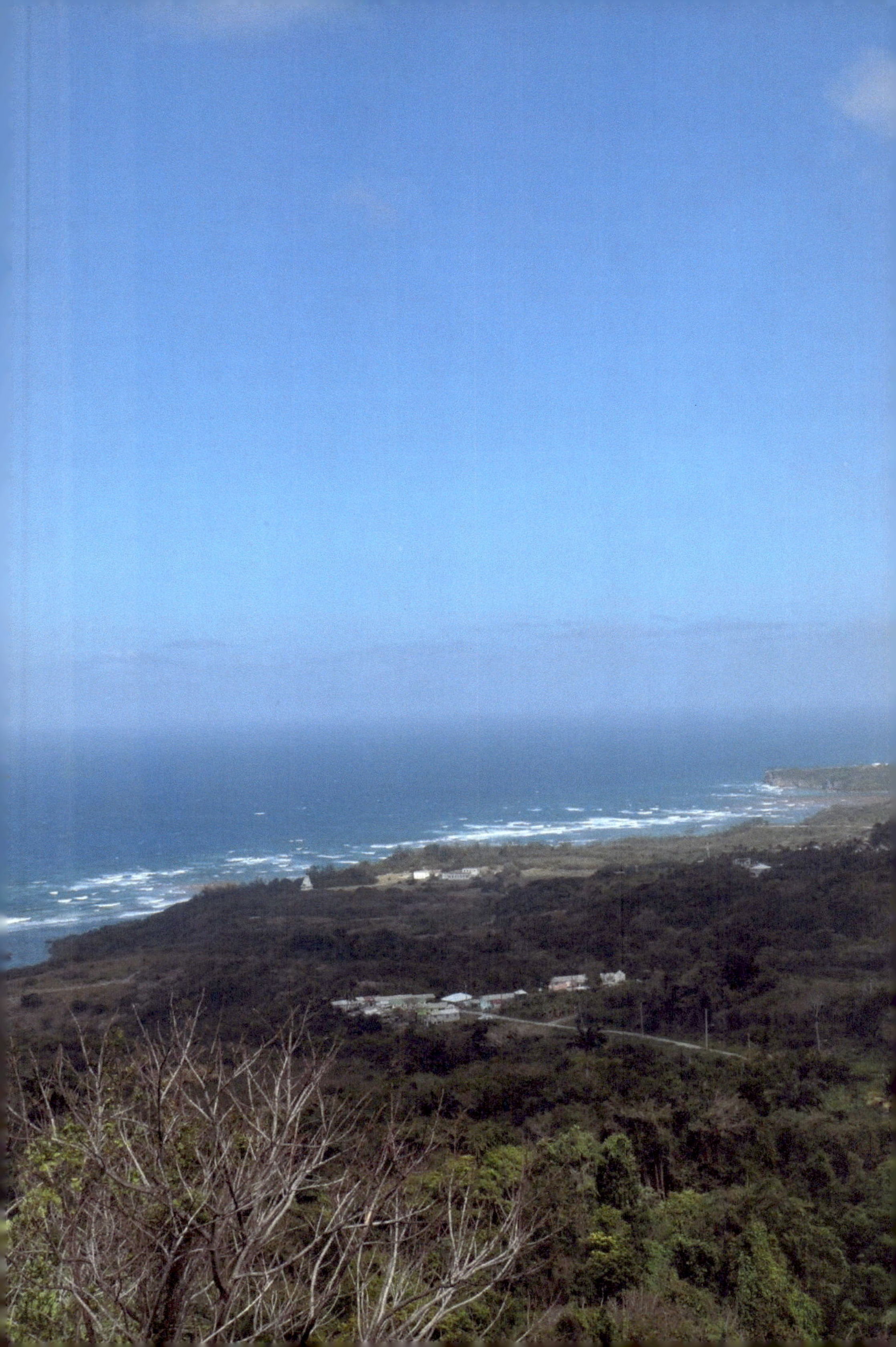

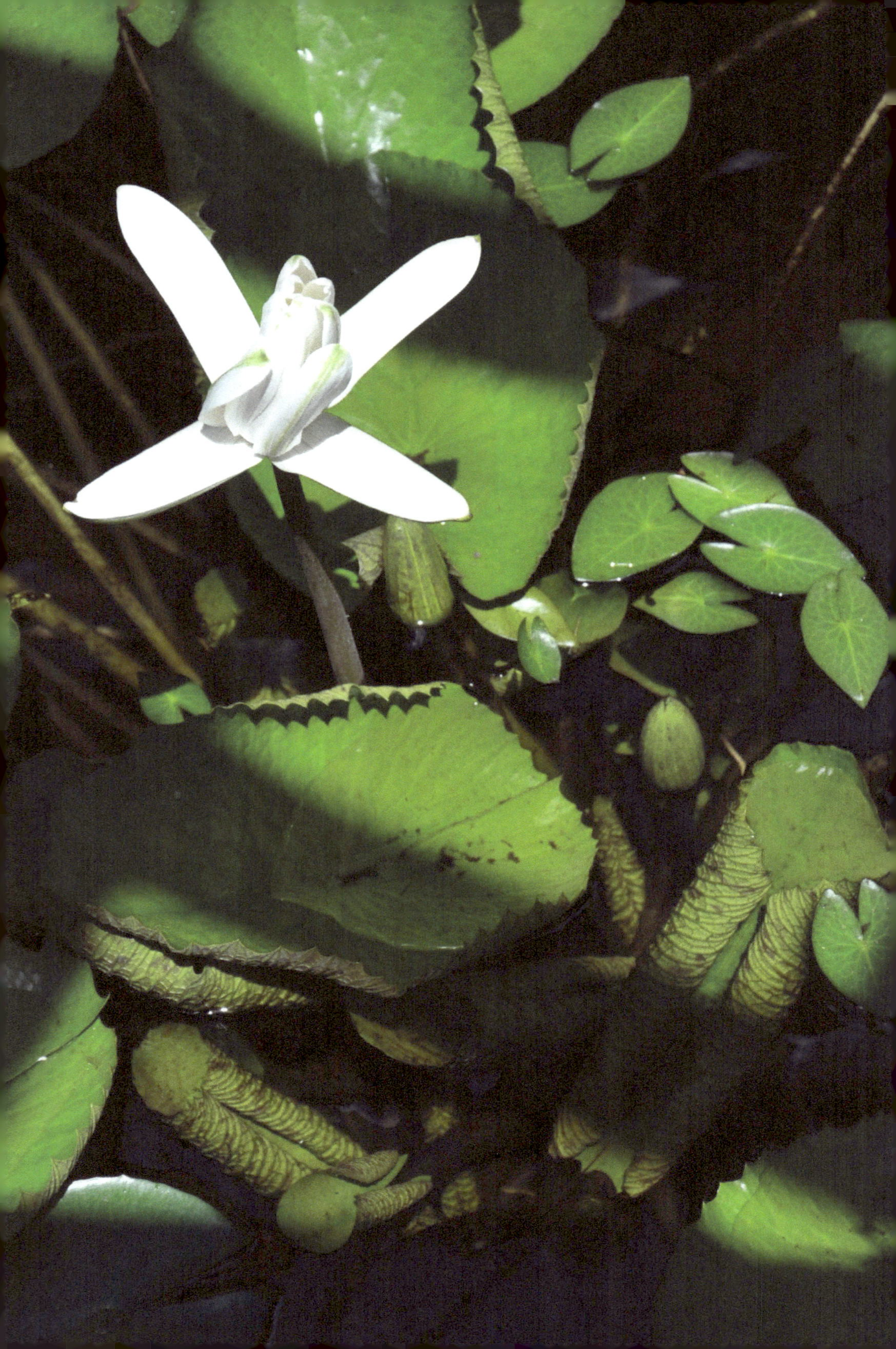

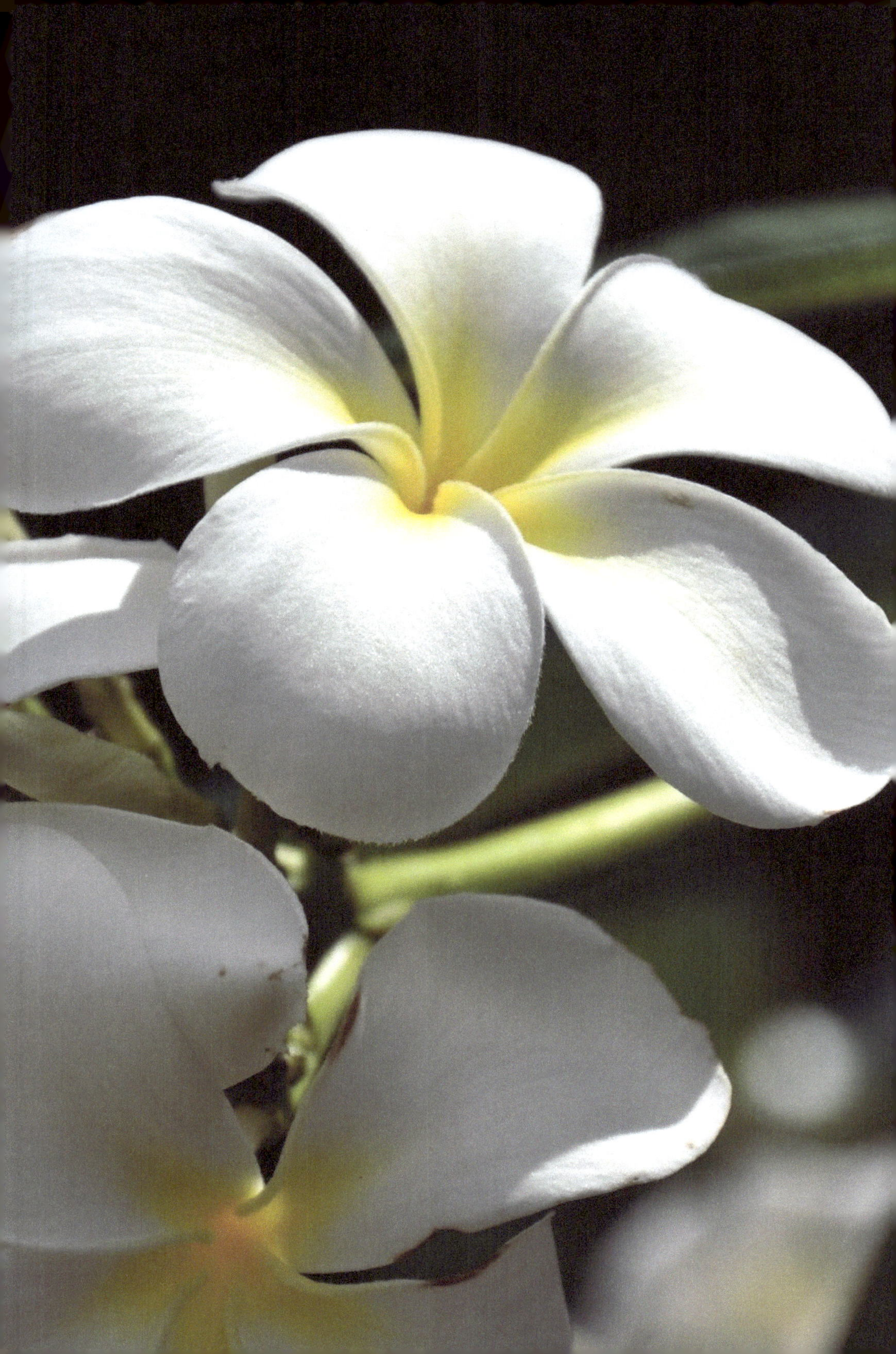

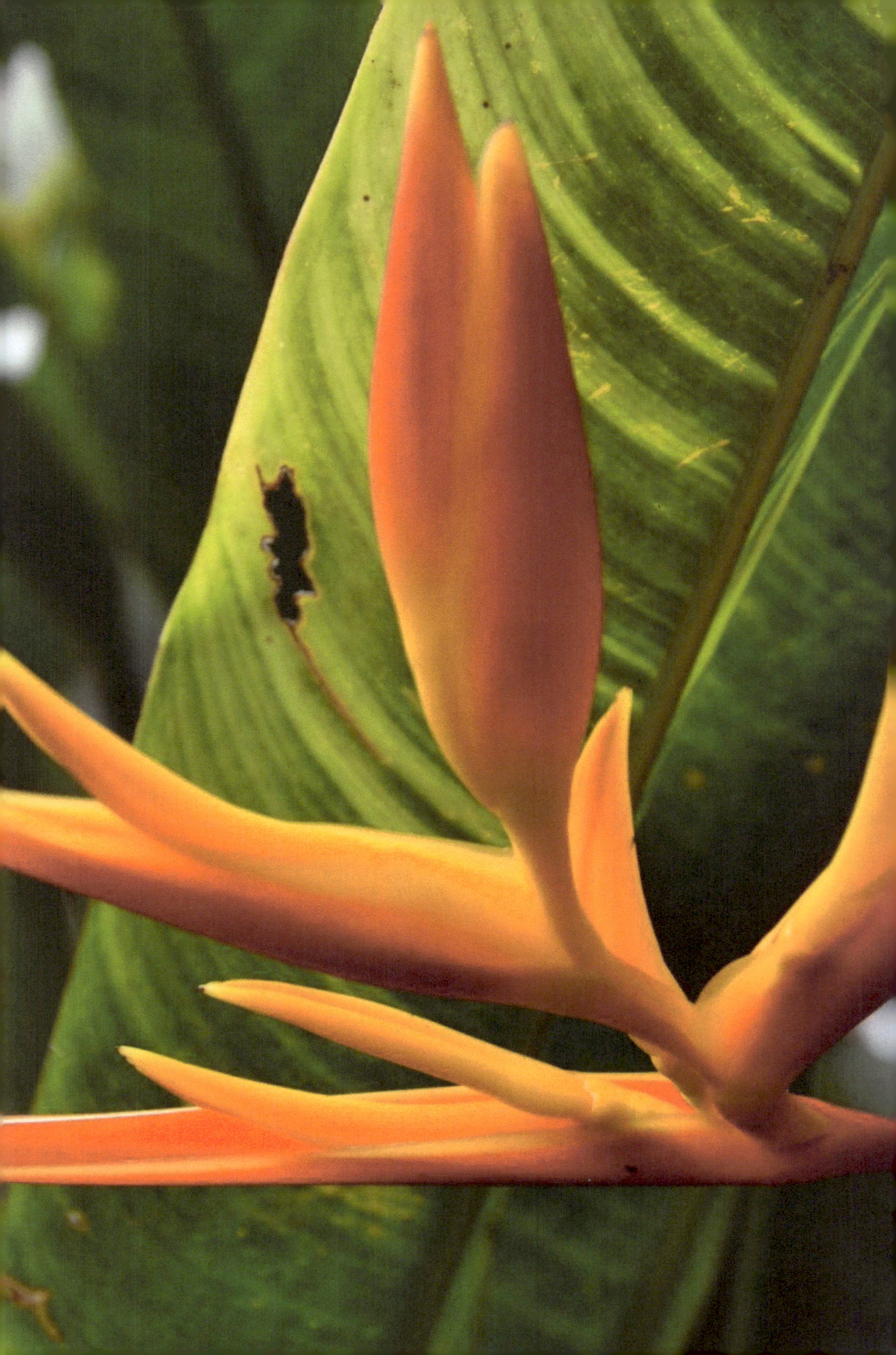

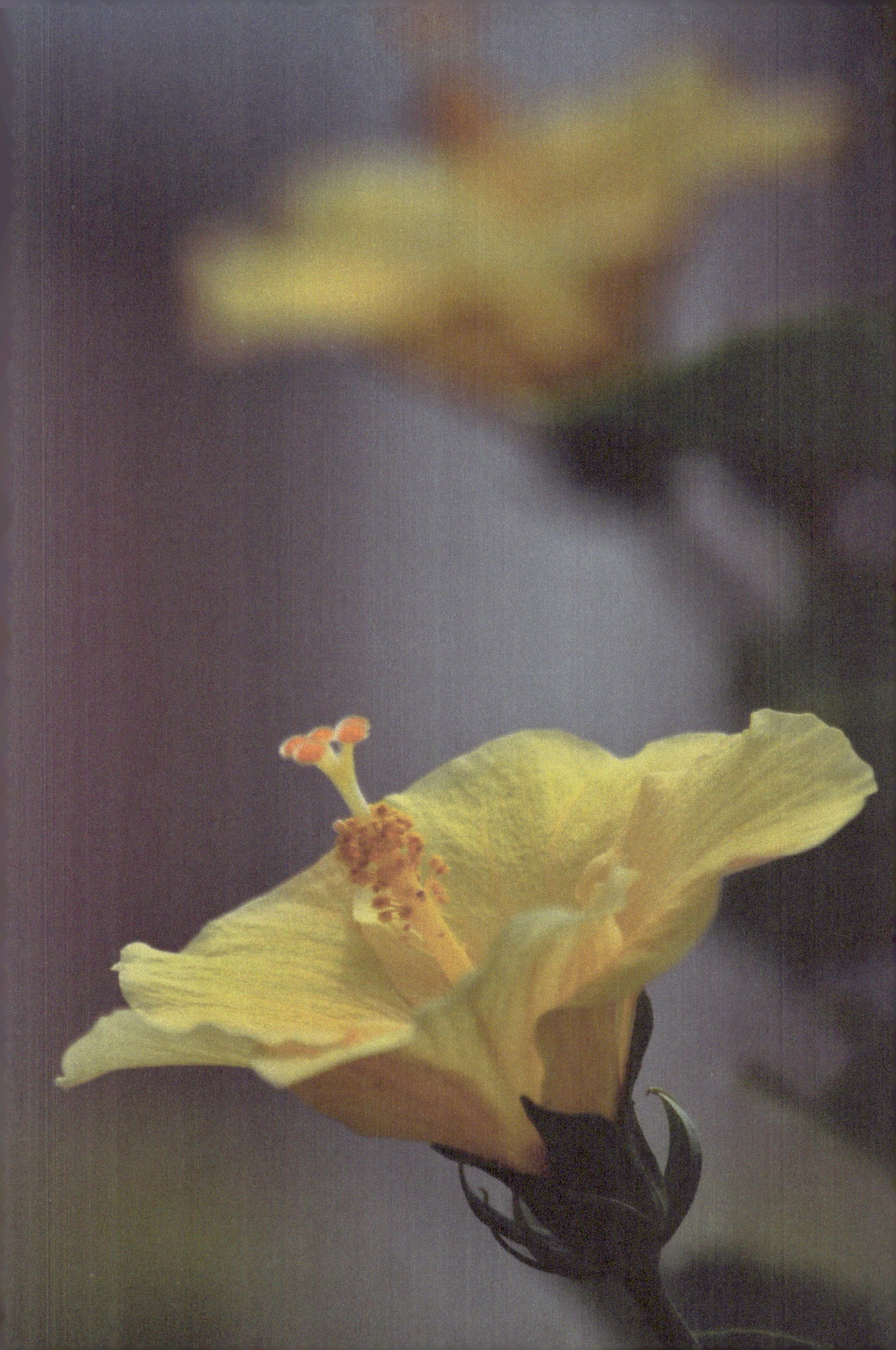

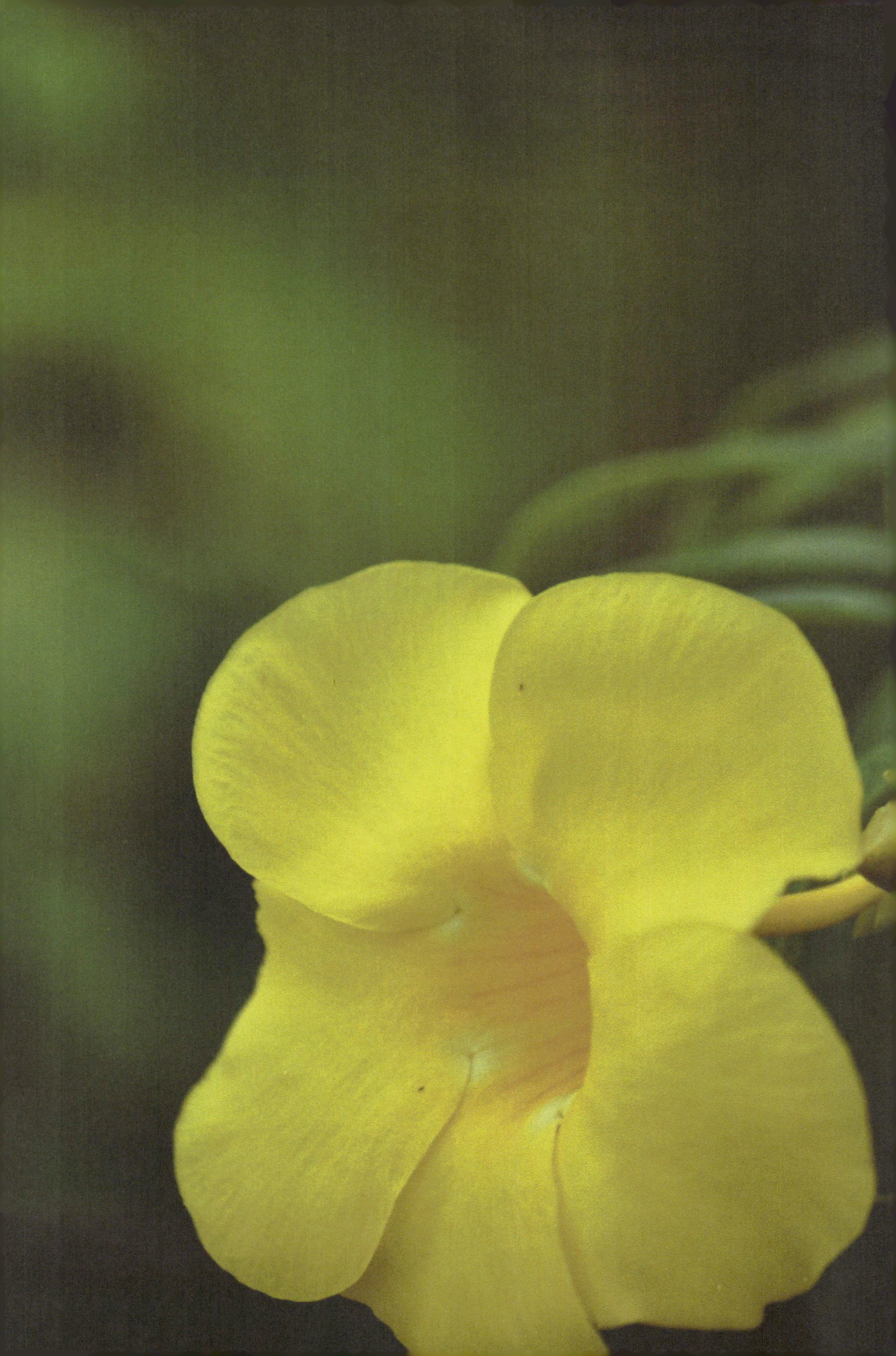

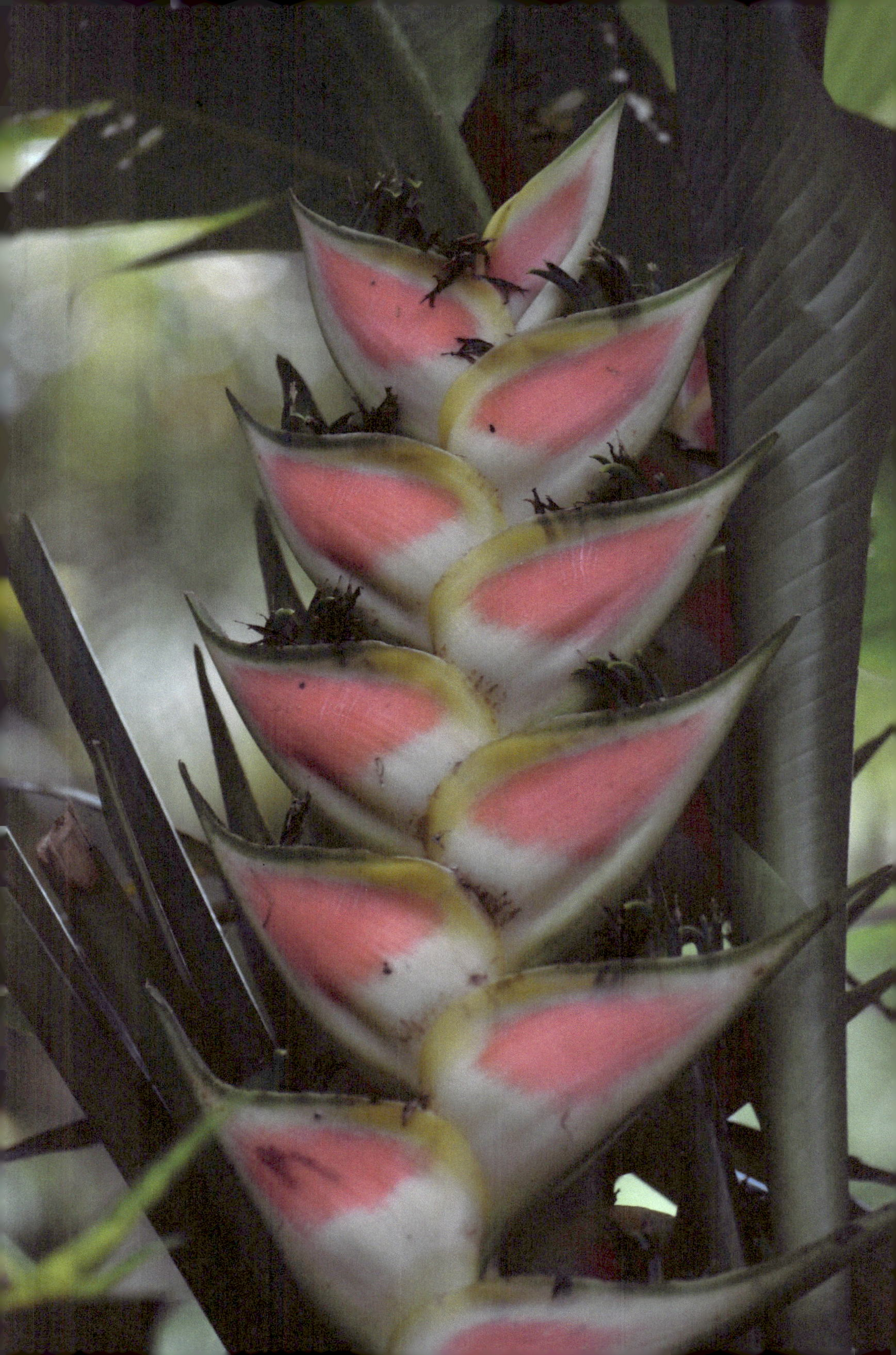

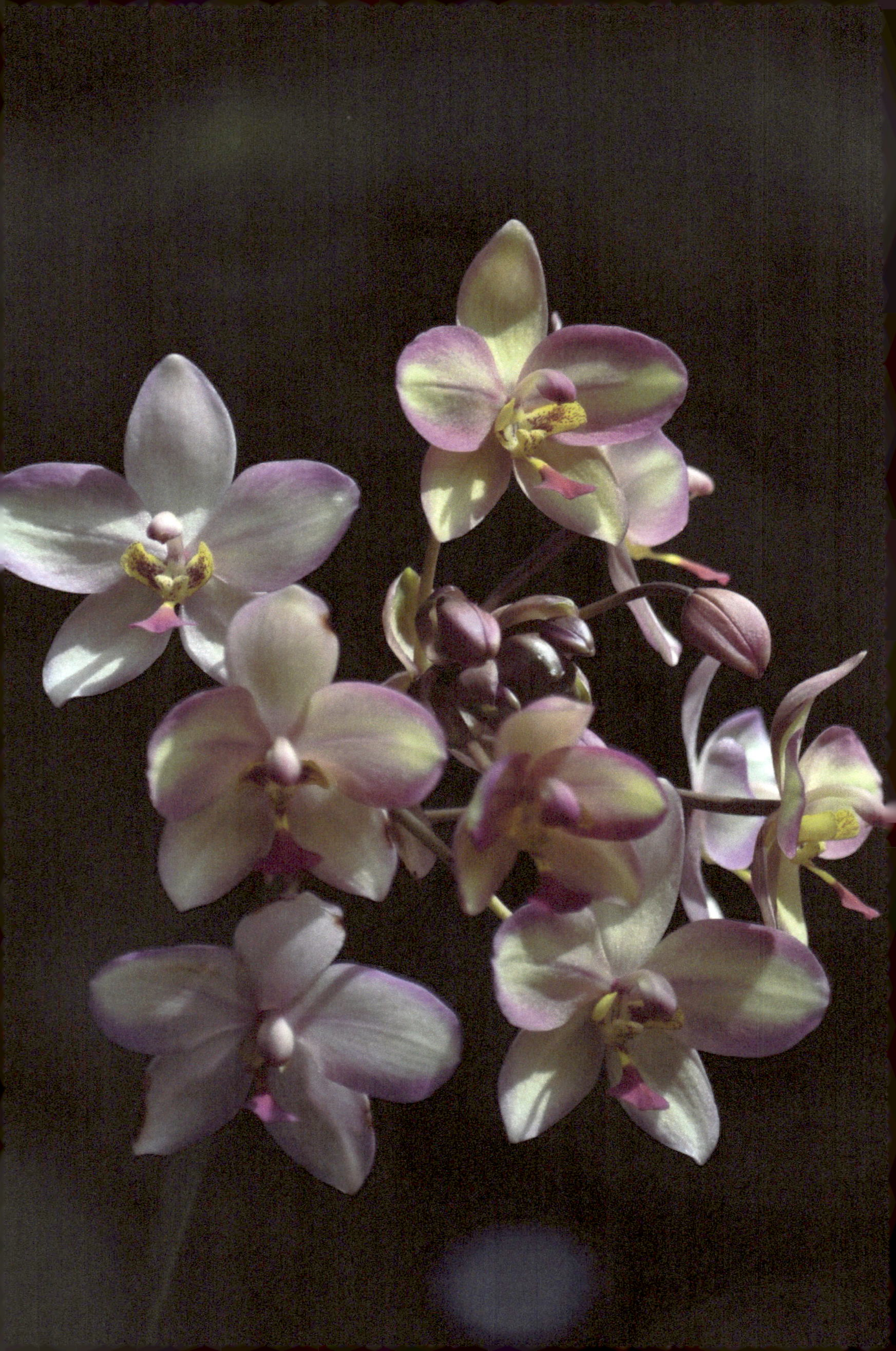

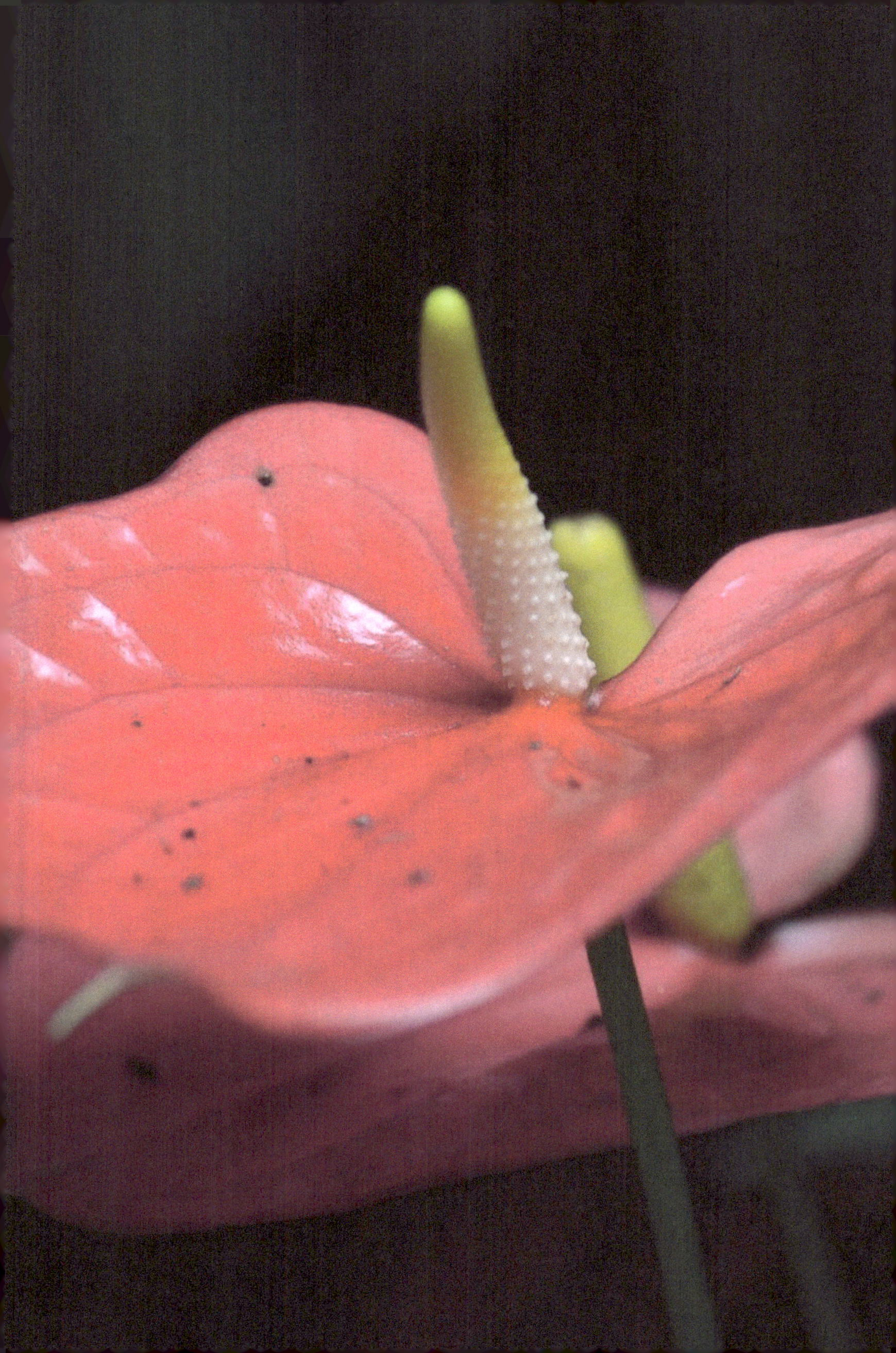

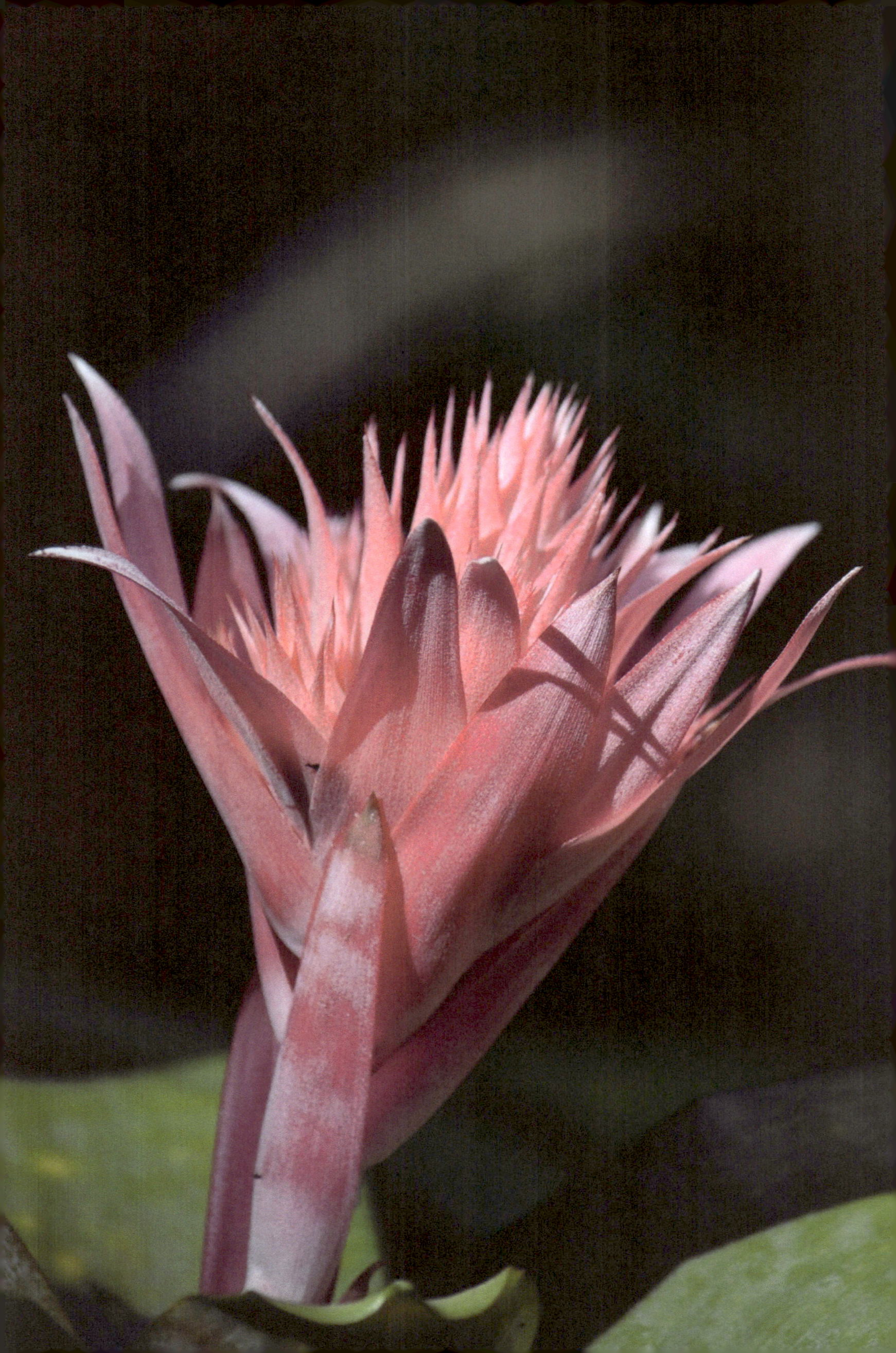

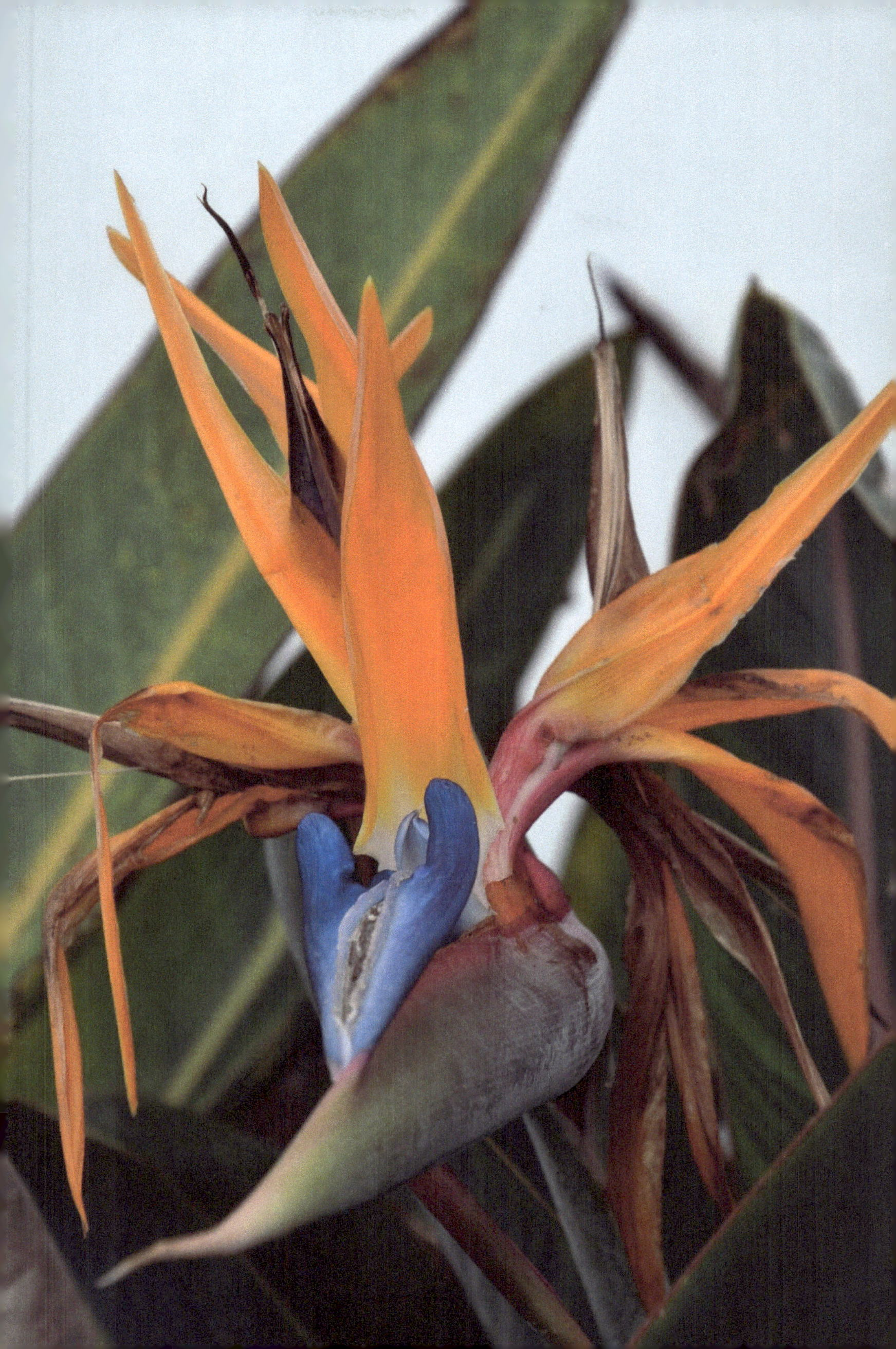

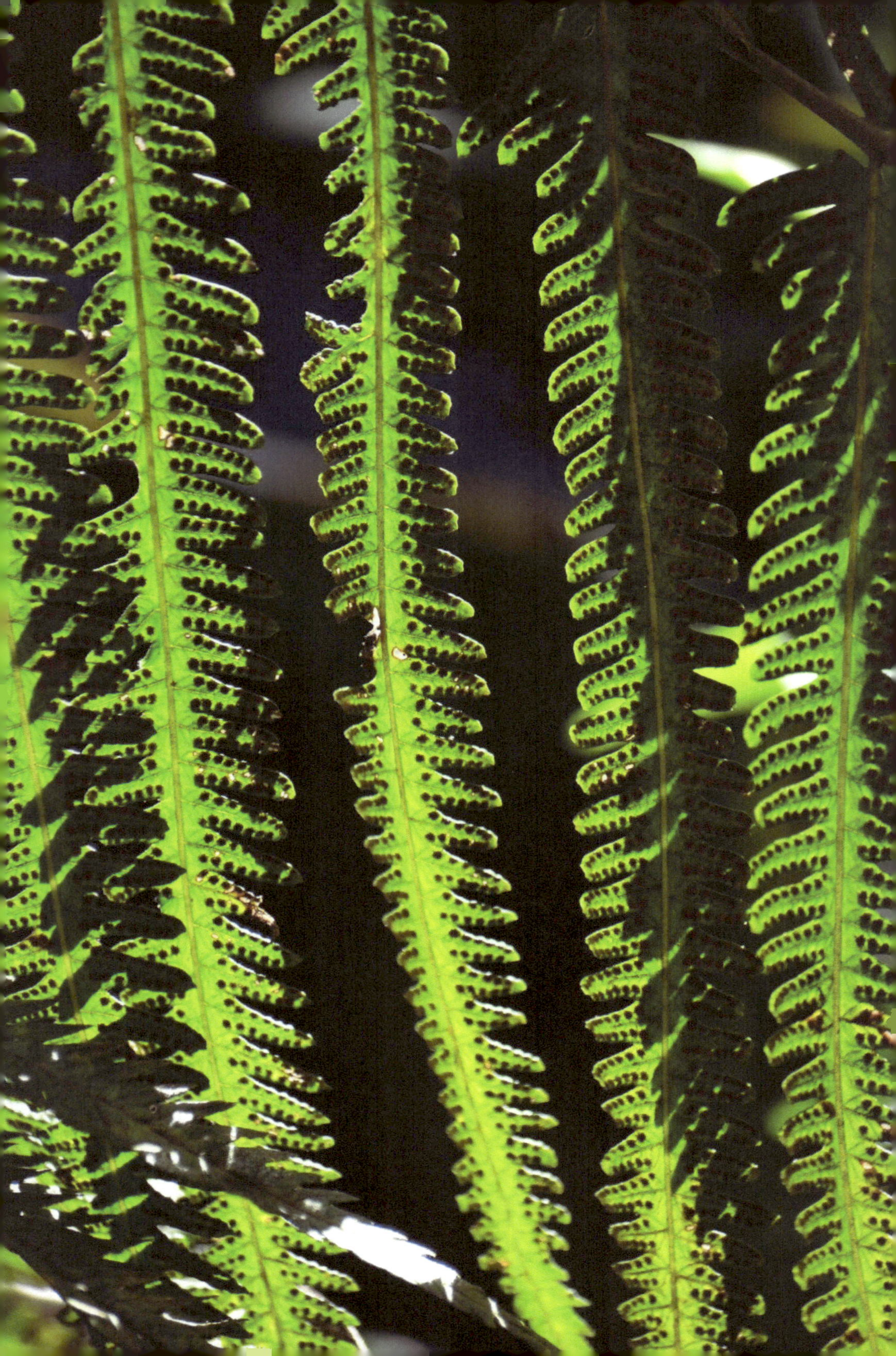

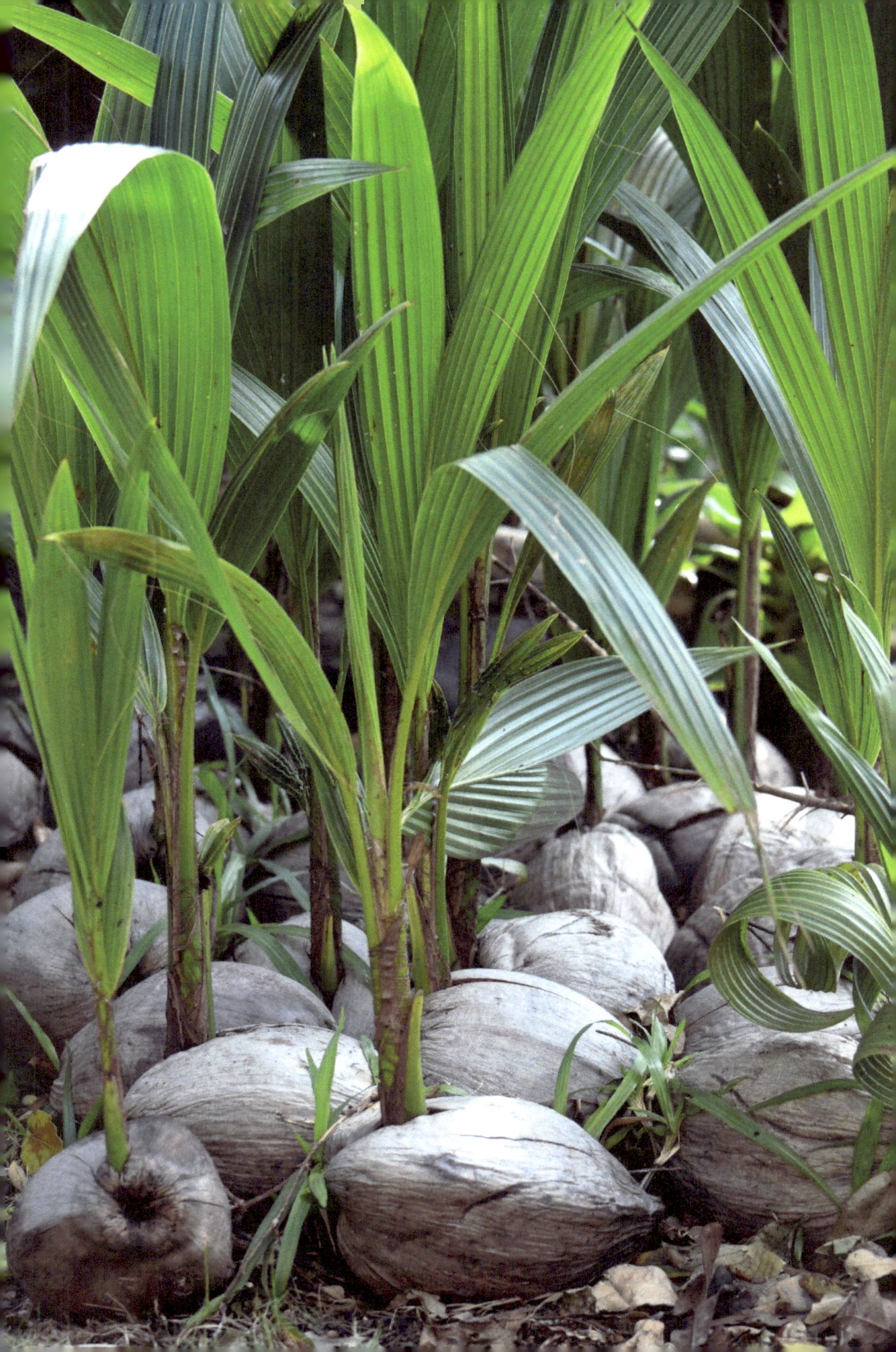

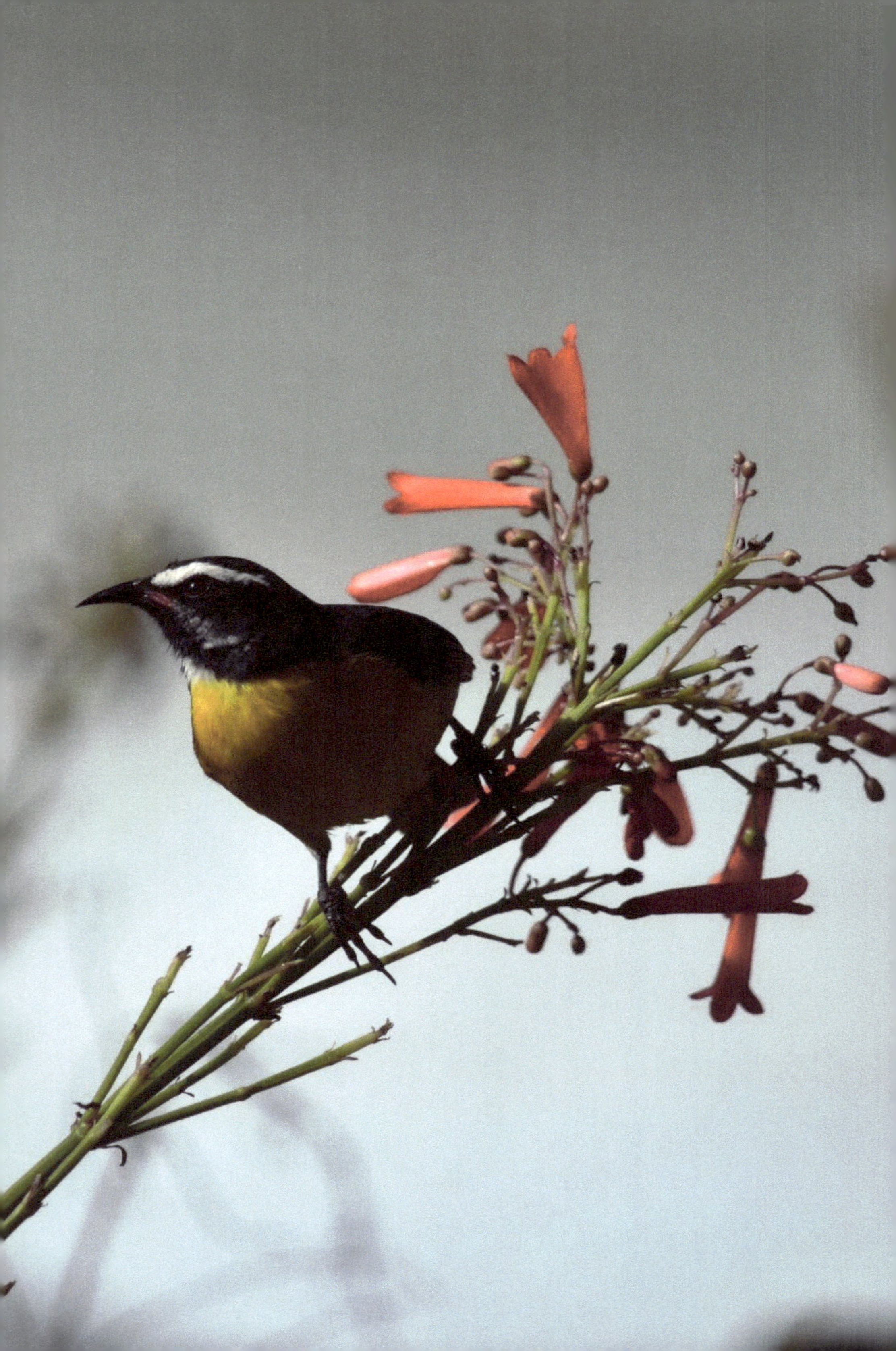

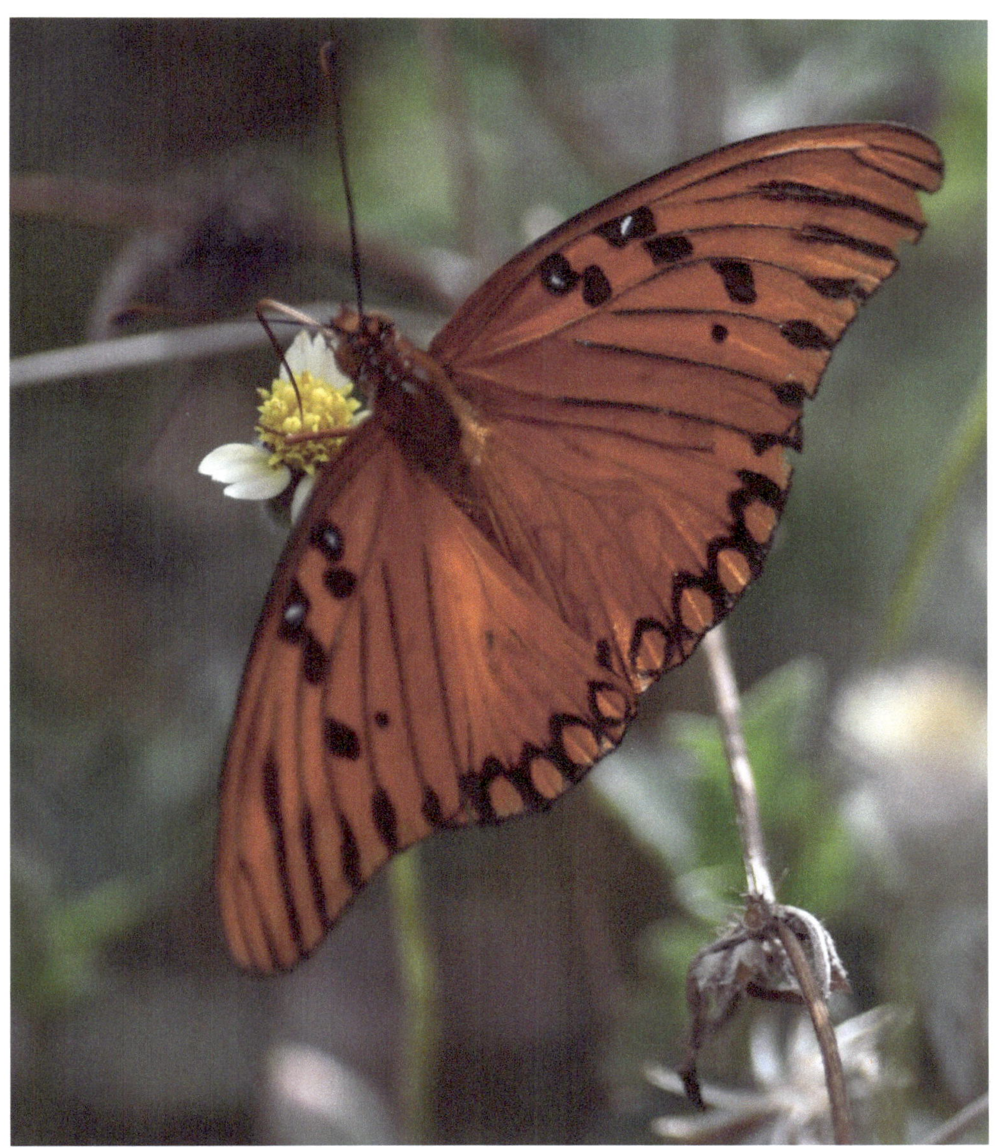

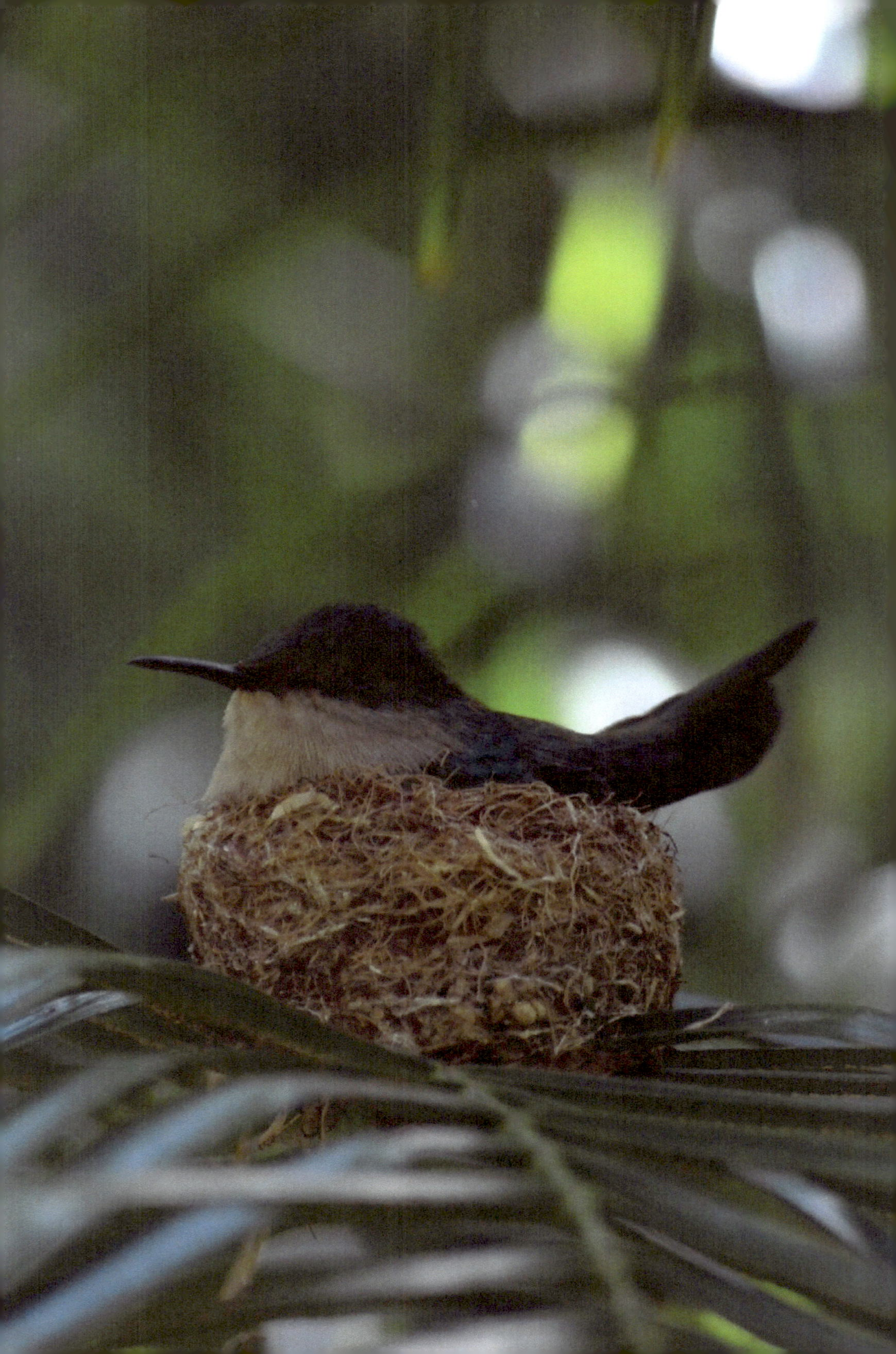

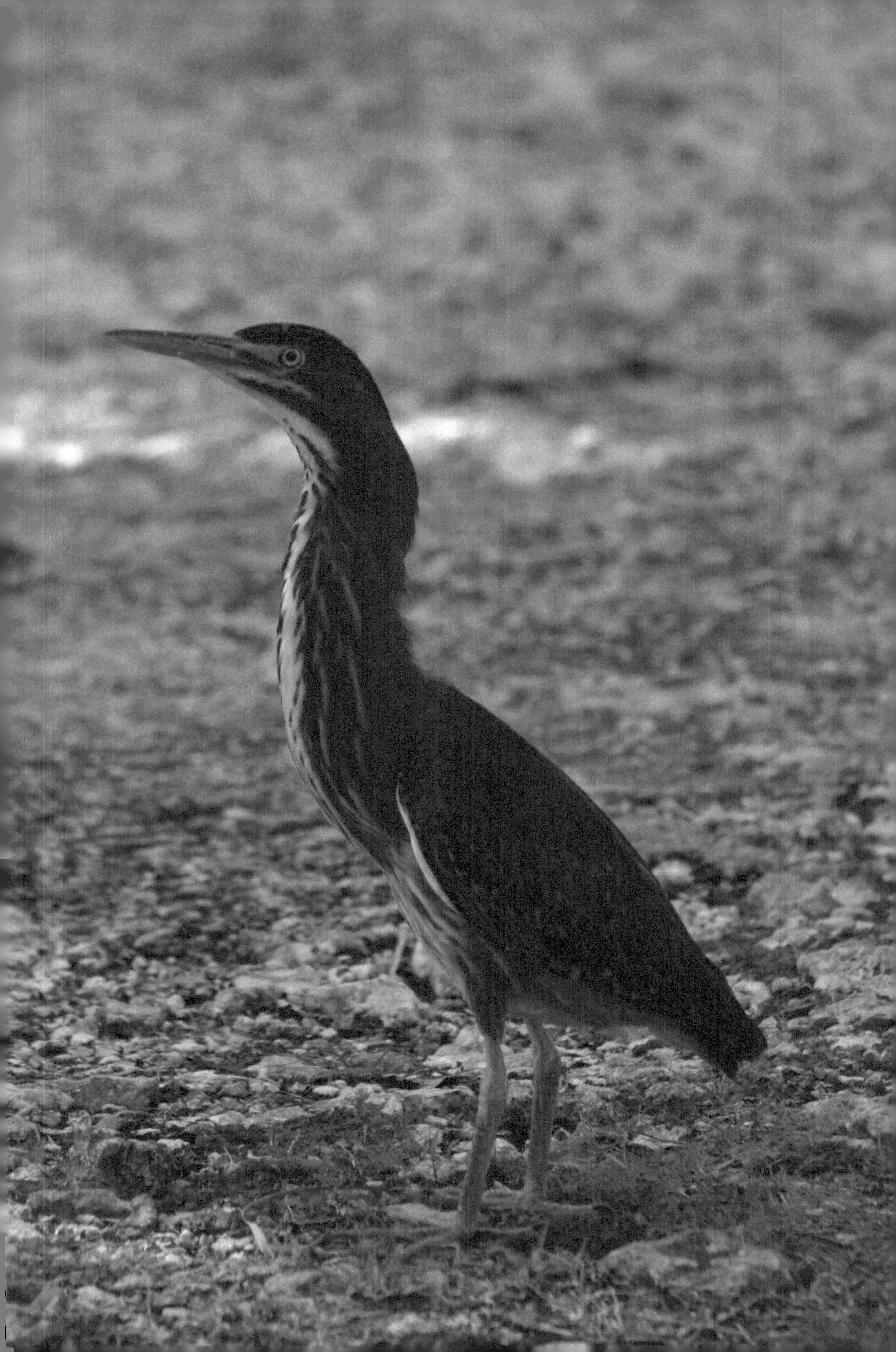

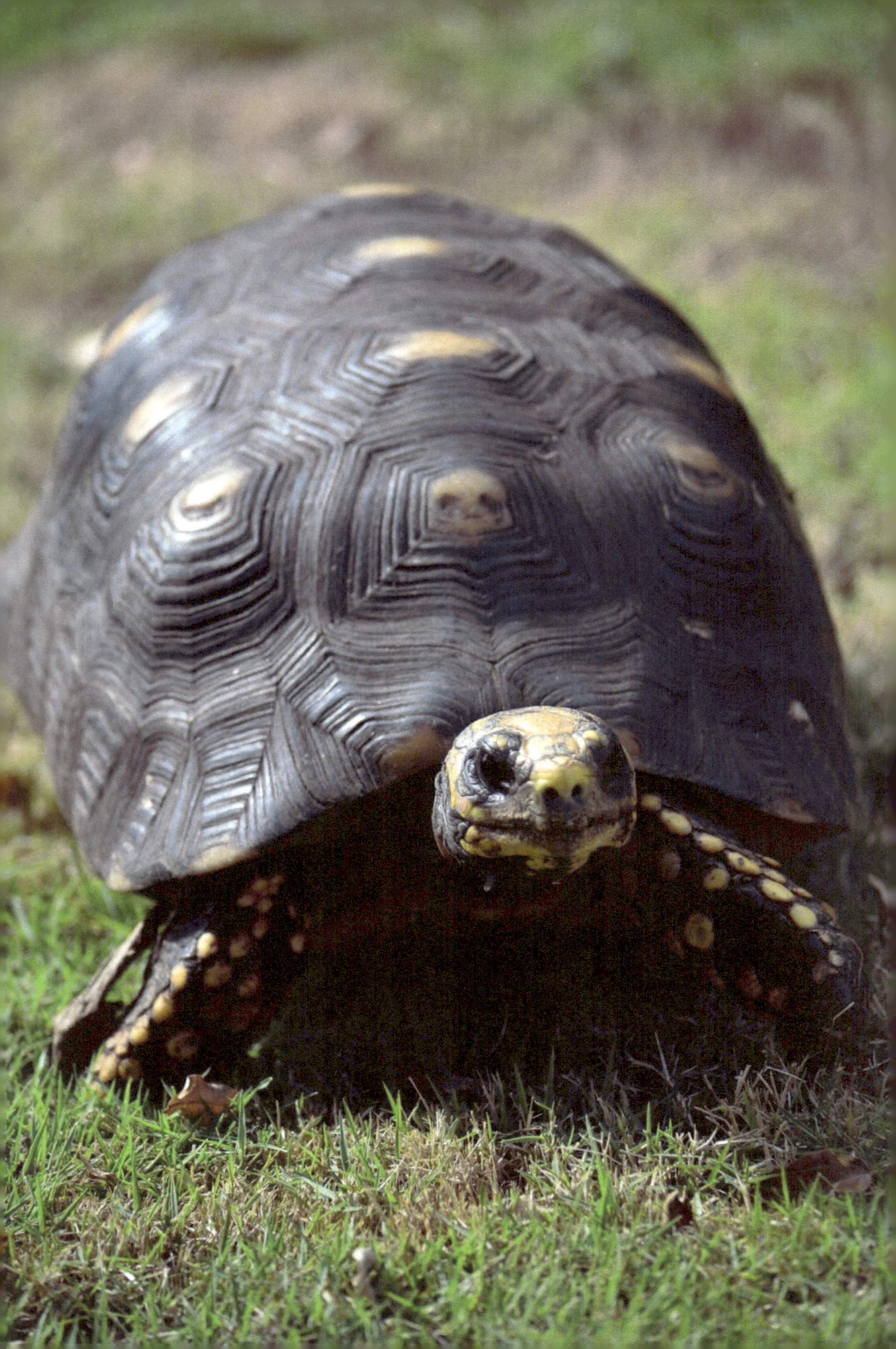

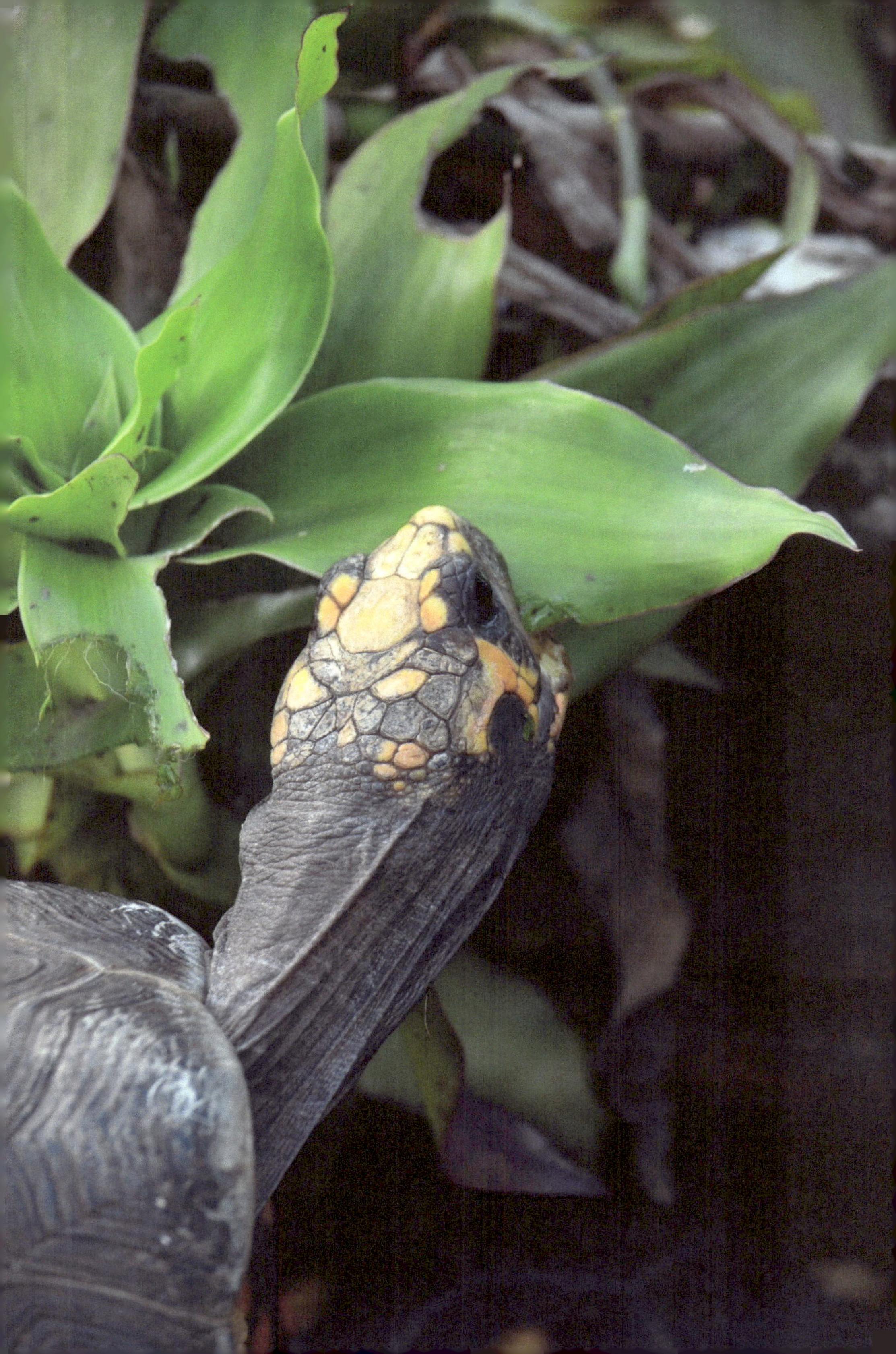

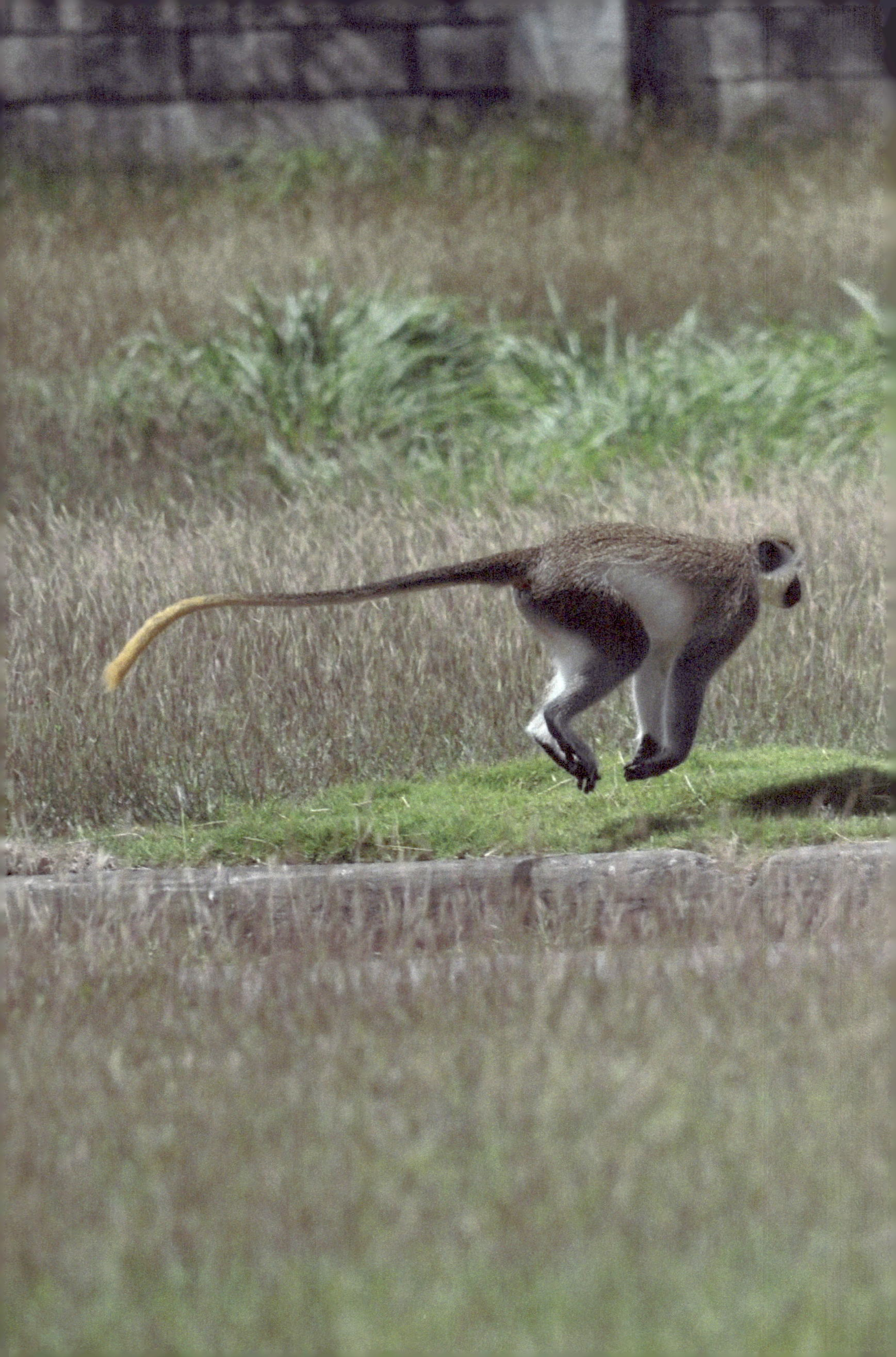

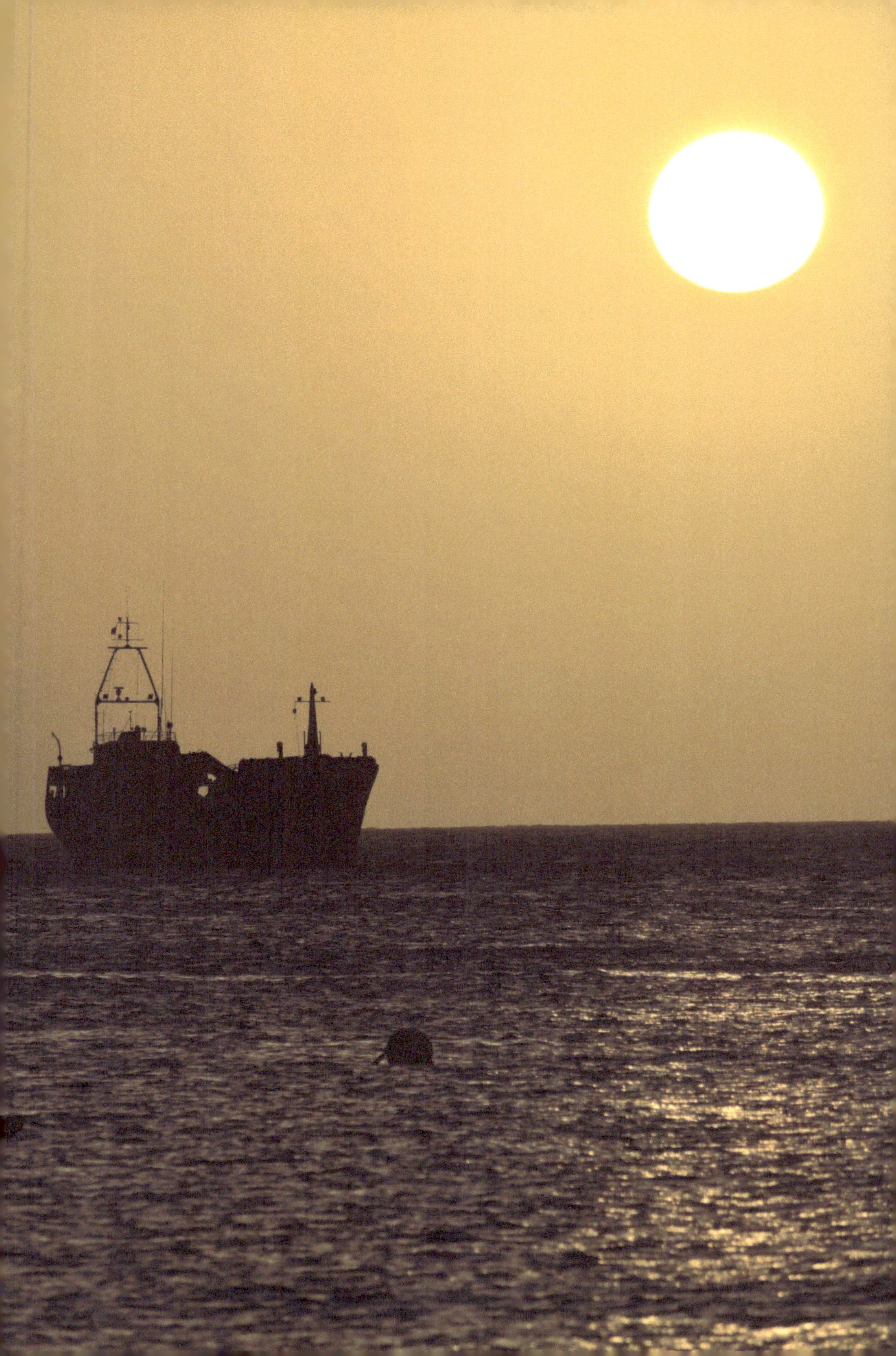

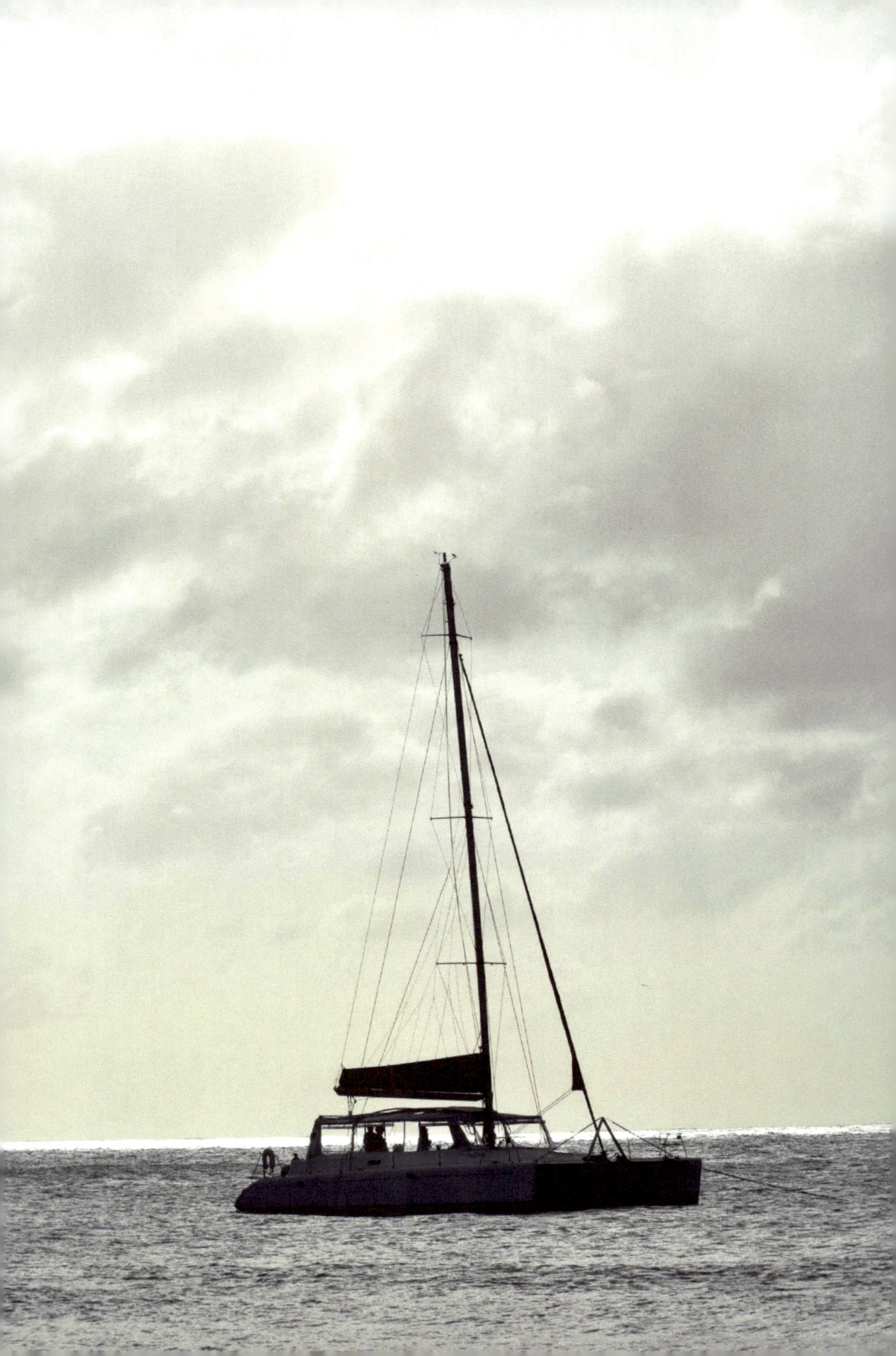

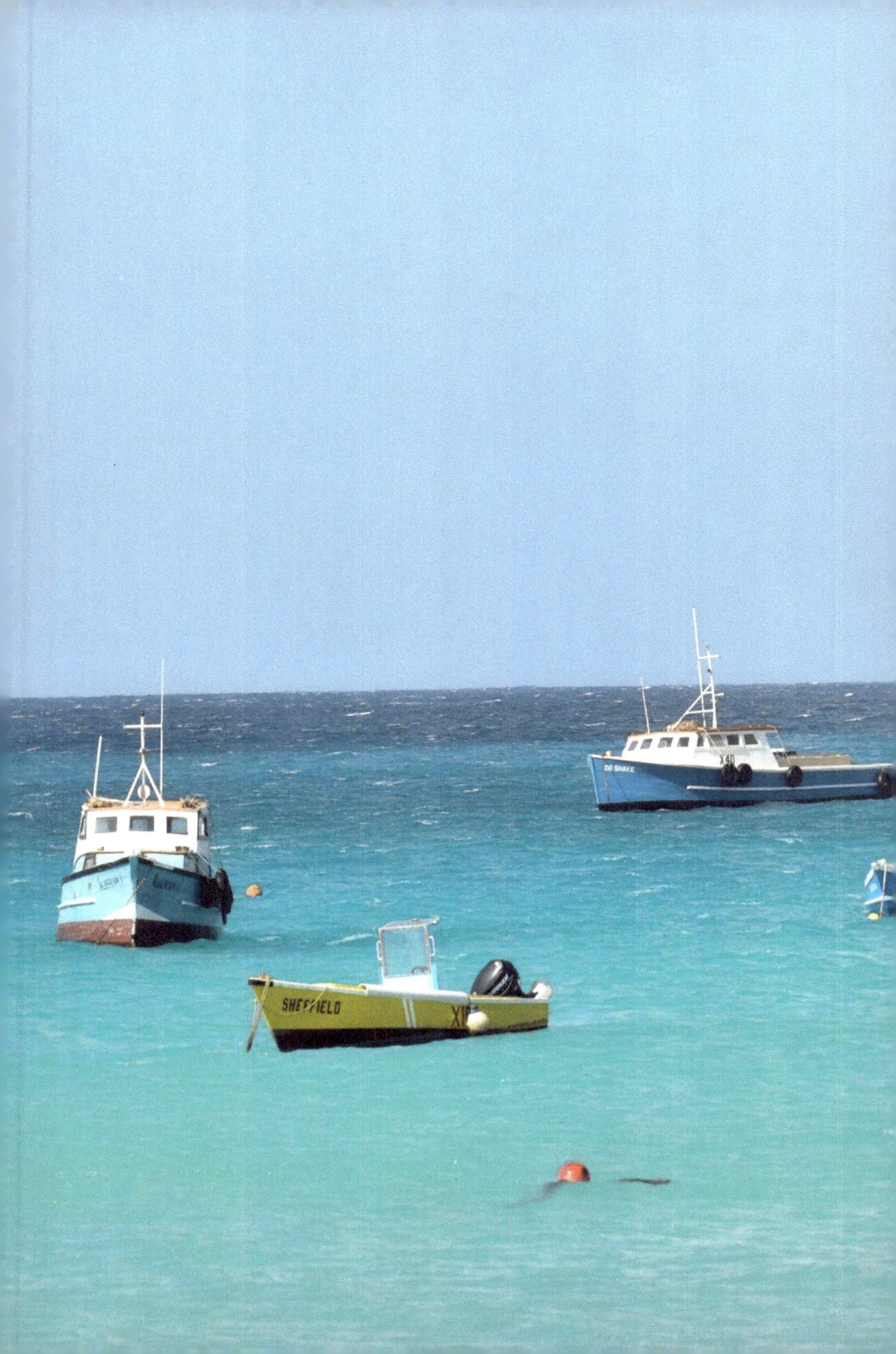
DE SNAKE
X40
SHEFFIELD

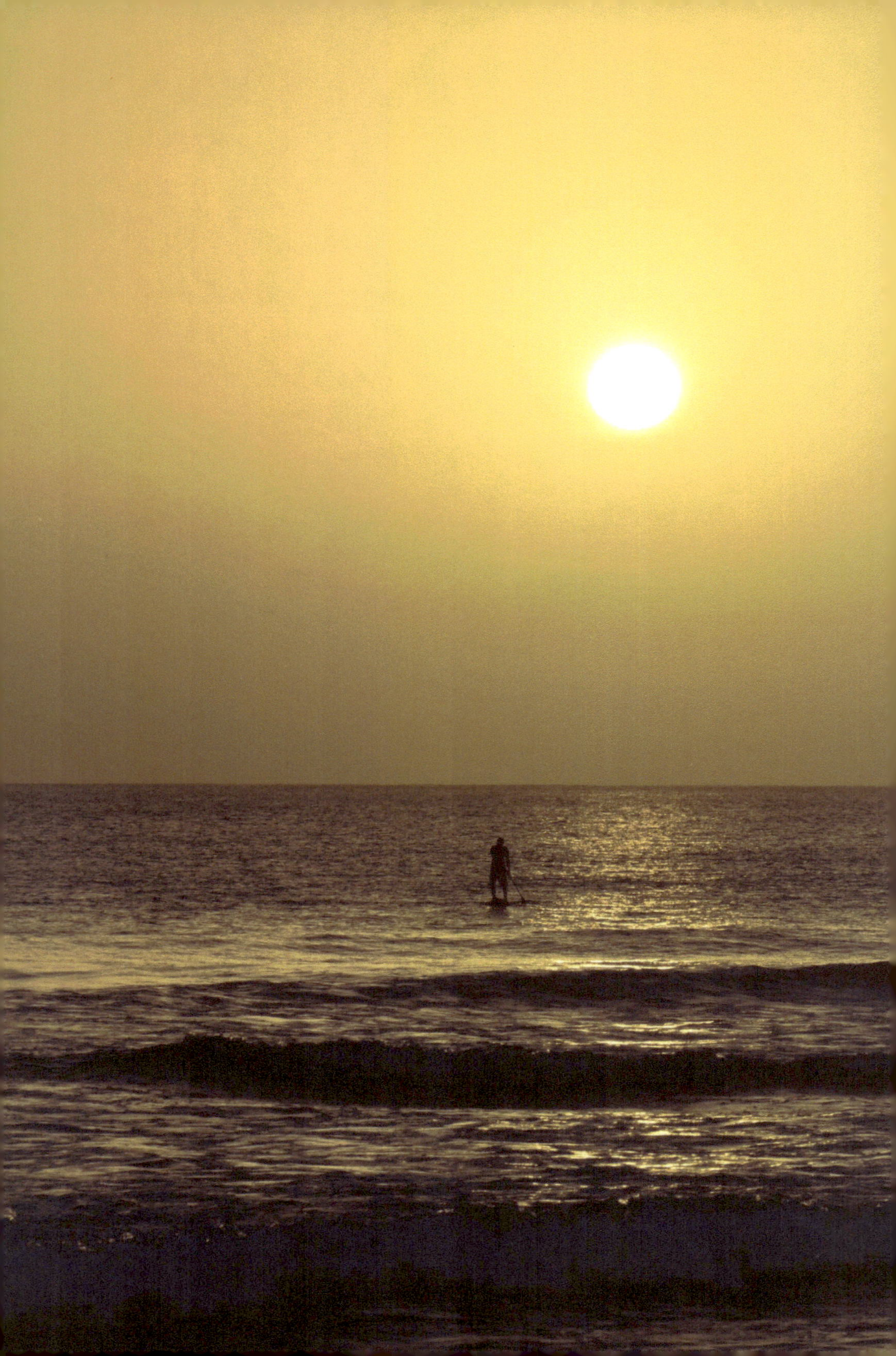